Always Hungry

Always Hungry

How I Lost the Weight and Found Myself

Jane McGuinness

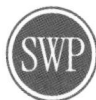

SWP

SHE WRITES PRESS

Published in 2025 by
She Writes Press, an imprint of The Stable Book Group

32 Court Street, Suite 2109
Brooklyn, NY 11201
https://shewritespress.com
Library of Congress Control Number: 2025909424
ISBN: 978-1-64742-986-7
eISBN: 978-1-64742-987-4

Interior Designer: Andrea Reider

Printed in the United States
Names and identifying characteristics have been changed to protect the privacy of certain individuals.

For CB, Emily, and Alex,
always,
and for Mum

broken hill

The two most powerful warriors
are patience and time.

—Leo Tolstoy

I ate to escape. To avoid. Sometimes to comfort. Rarely did I eat because I was actually hungry. I was eating in an attempt to satisfy so many different hungers, none of which were physical.

My name is Jane, and I am recovering from a lifetime of disordered eating.

Welcome to my story.

Sitting at Vancouver International Airport awaiting a delayed flight to Montana, the first of two that will return me to the arms of my lover and far away from my three beloved children, I ponder the granola bar in my backpack. Delayed flight. Bored. Food. A decades-old, automatic Pavlovian response, now unlearned. The old Jane would eat to escape this delay, to distract, to simply pass the time while I await the plane that is still not yet here. The Jane who is healing recognizes that I'm not actually hungry for food, and that my stomach has zero desire for a chocolate almond bar. So, I decide to read a book instead.

So often we eat to be somewhere else. It's a temporary and effective solution—for five seconds. But it's flawed. Unhelpful. And when repeated on a daily basis, wildly unhealthy for our physical and mental health. Do I want to be stuck in an airport? No. Will eating the granola bar change that? No.

Ultimately, an eating disorder is a life disorder. I look at photos of my former self, horrified. Mortified that I could ever let myself get so big. I still struggle to look at these pictures. Only now I look with compassion and feel a sadness for the girl who was not coping with life. She was struggling. Struggling with a lack of self-worth, shame, feelings of inadequacy. Struggling with three small children, one with autism (undiagnosed at the time). Struggling with no immediate family support and a husband who worked long hours and traveled. And so, she escaped. Her chosen escape, dangerously close by, was the kitchen.

As I sit here half-listening to the announcements overhead, I wonder, *Just when did flying become waiting?* I shift from one uncomfortable airport seat to another in order to access that most useful of all airport installations: the power outlet. Doing so, I ponder the insanity that is our modern world, and I'm struck by an idea: I've decided that it's high time we start handing out awards for stupidity on flights. Much like the Darwin Awards—those hilarious collections of ineptitude where many people of questionable intelligence successfully eliminate themselves from the gene pool—their (often) premature expiration eliminates any further chance that these defective genes could be passed on to offspring. Let's face it: The world isn't short on stupidity, and recipients truly earn those awards by virtue of their ultimate sacrifice. Quite frankly, it's time for the aeronautical equivalent. Frequent Flyers? Frequent Fuckwits is more like it. FF, yes?

And without further ado, let me begin with the first two nominations. Both contenders for an FF award go to my fellow passengers on a long-haul Montreal to Athens flight in 2022. First problem: The flight was full. Second problem: Everyone had carry-on (few people trusting to check a bag post pandemic).

Now the third problem was caused by two individuals and our inaugural FF nominees. Nominee 1, for some inexplicable reason, had decided to take a huge chunk of desperately needed overhead bin space for a supersized Costco-branded box of dried fruit, leaving several nearby passengers with no space for their roller bags. The mind boggles. Was this gentleman not aware that dried fruit was available on the Greek mainland? Did he have some kind of internal blockage and require this mountain of fiber? Or was he simply trying to win an FF on the day in question?

Now Nominee 2 was a different kettle of fish altogether. Wildly overdressed (and over-Botoxed), this woman informed everyone in the vicinity, quite loudly, that she was attending a wedding in Greece and required an entire overhead bin for herself to lie flat a dress, hat, and breakable wedding gift. We all looked on with expressions ranging from bewilderment to anger. As for myself, my bemused expression quickly turned to annoyance. (Again, several nearby passengers were left with no space for their bags). A heated debate ensued with a diplomatic young flight attendant who enquired, "Could you possibly put this at your feet, ma'am? Under the seat in front?"

"Oh no! This is *very* breakable! And my dress is for the wedding!" she told us all. I looked up. A good three-quarters of the overhead bin above the horizontally laying dress was one huge void. "My dress could be crushed!"

To be clear, she was quite serious about this impending disaster. To me, the greater disaster was that entitled people like this exist. This entitled member of the human race clearly didn't give a shit that she had commandeered an entire overhead bin for herself. Did she think she was in first class? She was certainly dressed like someone who was off to watch polo for the day. All that was lacking was the mimosa. Should someone bring her one? At the very least she might have calmed the fuck down about her precious, breakable (and wildly excessive) carry-on.

And why did they let her board with so much carry-on? So many unanswered questions. Astonished at her lack of consideration for others, the inaugural FF award went to the overdressed lady in 37G (pause for applause). Her long-suffering husband looked on in resignation. It was clear that he'd experienced decades of this Karen-behavior shitshow, God help him.

I now find that being on the lookout for future FF nominees while in the portal is a surprising amount of fun. And it certainly passes the time while moving from point A to B. Now the FF awards can't possibly be as illustrious as the Darwin Awards, because in the case of our hapless FFs, they aren't actually removing themselves from the gene pool. Oh no! These special individuals live to fly another day, only one Expedia booking away from inconveniencing a new group of weary travelers. It doesn't seem fair that they get their own book. Not yet anyway. Perhaps a dedicated blog space for our FFs? I shall give this further thought.

"Jane, get out of the fridge!" A common refrain from my mother.

"But I'm *bored!*" My usual response.

And I was bored. An outback Australian mining town in the mid-1980s didn't offer up a lot in the way of entertainment for a tween, which probably went part way to explaining the higher-than-national average teen pregnancy rate. Nevertheless, I wasn't standing with the refrigerator door wide open due to boredom, despite my protest. I was looking for answers that were never going to be found between the Vegemite and the iceberg lettuce. And why did every mother in the '80s think that salads required a base of the blandest ingredient on the planet? Ugh. No wonder it took me at least another decade to fall in love with greens.

And what was I looking for as I stood in the kitchen, day after day? Security? Love? Stability? A father I could actually rely on? Two parents whose days didn't start and end with shouting? Turns out it was all the above. And more.

"No." My father's response to everything. And it typically came before the question was asked. Homework help. Money for groceries at the corner store. A ride somewhere. "No."

Little did we know that my father had struggled with undiagnosed depression until his fiftieth year. Now with the right medication he's playing catch up, and he's trying. For that I am patient. Of course, he remains an emotional eater. The apple really doesn't fall far from the tree, does it?

He'd tell my mother, "Later on. I'll get to it!"

"Later on."

Ron: my mother's shorthand. Ron never did get to most of what needed doing. The chopping of the firewood and the mowing of the lawn fell to her after the school day was done. I took over the lawncare for the most part when I was old enough.

"Wear closed shoes." Her sage advice.

I did.

As for Ron, I don't know where the fuck he was, but he never did get to everything.

High school was dreadful. My attendance was excellent, in part due to my hunger for knowledge and a yearning to discover everything that existed outside of the ignorant, small-minded town of my youth. Desperate to escape, my attendance was also excellent because my mother would have it no other way. Her job as the local high school math teacher put food on the table and ensured that we always knew the value and importance of education. And besides, I was smart enough to know that good grades were my one-way ticket out of this shithole of a town.

I had little in common with my peers. While they were busy getting drunk and pregnant, I was at the local library. While lost in the stacks, hungry to submerse myself in another world, my peers were attempting to escape into a drunken stupor, weekend after weekend. Someone rather industrious, with just the right disregard for the law, had the rather brilliant idea to provide a dial-a-beer service. Easy money. No one had to drive anywhere (clearly) or hope their fake ID passed inspection at the local bottle shop. Oh no, they just needed to pick up the telephone. Yes, in those days it was still plugged into the wall. If you were lucky, your parents bought one of the cordless brick styles we saw on US sitcoms. We were still years away from cell phones. To this day I wonder if the police simply turned a blind eye . . . or perhaps benefited from this hustle?

The boys would have some sketchy, homemade fake ID and attempt to lower their voices. I recall one faintly amusing boy stuffing a pair of socks down the front of his jeans. Now, apart from being no doubt uncomfortable, I don't see how this could have possibly made the young chap appear any older. He was all of fifteen, and his voice had yet to break. Who was he kidding? Fortunately for young Jason, he didn't have to kid anyone. The driver happily took his cash in exchange for twenty-four cans of beer. Such was Broken Hill in the '90s. Bored kids. Drinking. Sex. I stuck to eating. After all, my mother was the local math teacher. I was about as far from cool as anyone could get. I was in no danger of becoming popular, and I've come to the conclusion that this was a very good thing. No one wants to peak in high school, trust me. Remember the bullied kids, often labeled weird, sometimes brilliant? The ones to watch. For the cool kids of my youth, it was typically a slow, downward trajectory beginning soon after graduation.

The library was deliciously cool on a hot day, thanks to the industrial AC, and calm where home was not. In retrospect, I was likely craving the peaceful, orderly refuge that this old rendered brick building provided. I'd also craved a swimming pool and would often fantasize about the backyard pool that we could build. Between books, I'd while away the hours sketching rather impressive architectural drawings for a pool that would never be built. We simply didn't have the money, and even if we did, who would have maintained it? My mother was busy chopping firewood and playing golf in her precious free time, and my father was often simply missing, and anyway, his answer was always no. I was stuck.

Being the rather determined teenager that I was, I decided one scorching Aussie summer that it was time to take matters into my own hands. Off to the shed I went. As luck would have it, not only did my father rarely get to anything, he also rarely tidied the shed. As a result, there were decades of treasures to be found among the broken-down odds and ends. Rusted old rabbit traps hung from the rafters, relics of my late grandfather's former pastime. The scent of grease and petrol. The dug-out pit for working on cars, covered with railway sleepers, the depths of which always scared me just a little. My best friend of thirty-plus years, Kellie, remembers with fondness the broken-down forklift. Why did we have it, you ask? I still don't know. My father was getting to it.

And in the meantime, I was getting to work. Old car tires, huge swathes of thick black plastic, and an assortment of bricks would do the trick. And yes, they did! For about three days I had the most impressive (and entirely free) above ground pool the town had ever seen. Of course, the following week I also had the most impressive ear infection that the doctor had ever seen. Chlorine was an afterthought. As were the spiders. Up until that point, they were happily residing in that small mountain of black plastic. I recall my scream that could wake the dead when I inadvertently disturbed a family of redbacks who were less than impressed with my construction project. Looking back, it's a wonder I survived my childhood at all.

I was terribly self-conscious as a teen. Was everyone else just hiding their insecurities better than I? Perhaps. Boys teased. My voice, too loud.

"Hey, Jane, do you play the piano?" they hollered at me in the playground.

"Yes! Why?" Never one to be too quiet, I hollered right back. Laughter followed.

"You sound just like Rowlf from the Muppets!"

Well, this was news to me. Up until then anyway. In hindsight it could have been worse. To be fair, Rowlf, the piano-playing Muppet, was always my favorite of Jim Henson's motley crew, and like me, did have a fondness for the piano.

The comparison drawn due to my somewhat husky voice, I became quite embarrassed about the whole thing, despite my secret affection for Rowlf and his enthusiastic disposition. My voice, after all, was not something I had any control over. As a child people would ask my mother if I had a cold. It was only many years later that I learned that a husky voice is to some men quite alluring—think Lauren Becall in the '40s. Of course, I didn't know that yet. All I knew was that I was too big, too loud, and my voice just didn't have the same sweet soprano ring of my friends. And the underlying message? I wasn't good enough. I didn't fit in.

No one in my family fit in. Not my father with his out-spoken political views, not my overweight sister suffering with epilepsy, and certainly not me.

And so, I ate.

My comfort food wasn't the fast food of our modern era. Broken Hill didn't even have a McDonalds in the early '90s. Oh no. My waistline expanded in the kitchen as I stirred, sifted, and baked my way through my teens. Comfort on so many levels. But was I ever physically hungry? Rarely. I don't think I ever gave my body a chance to find out. Naturally, I became an excellent home chef. The problem was one of consumption.

The girls also teased. I recall the unpleasantness that was Amanda Wilson. Over our sewing machines in home economics one day, she was ruthless in her cruelty.

"Did you know that breasts are just pockets of fat, Jane? Did you know that?!"

Of course, Amanda was petite and rather flat-chested, and evidently despised the fact that I was already well-endowed. Now, the Wonder Bra had yet to make its way to Broken Hill to save her unfortunate flat chest, but she wore enough makeup and was pretty enough to think herself quite the teenage dream. Karma was twofold. I can't deny being delighted when, years later, she stopped with her illustrious gymnastics career, and her ass immediately started to widen.

The other delightful moment of karma was thanks to my perpetually stuffy nose. The dry, dusty climate of my hometown never did agree with me, much like the people. Both endured; neither enjoyed.

Kellie, while way cooler than I (read: "socially acceptable"), also wasn't immune from the cruelty that was Amanda Wilson. She still recalls Amanda's silent-but-deadly farts, always blamed on my dear best friend Kellie. I just thank God that I never sat close enough to be accused of the foul stench. I had enough to deal with. And I did always wonder . . . why Kellie didn't just move?! But I digress.

The scene was the school canteen line. Amanda with her smug, pert ass stood behind me. Passive-aggressive as always, she was telling me what I should and shouldn't be ordering for lunch if I did indeed want to lose weight. In any event it was particularly dusty that day, and my pockets were devoid of a tissue (I usually carried several). I will never forget the very moment I let out an uncontrollable sneeze, and the hugest, most disgusting stream of snot flew from my nose at an impressive rate and landed squarely on Amanda's forearm. It was at that moment that I knew that some kind of God existed. It was a certainty.

Sally Newton was less cruel, more of an amusing bully. Nevertheless, she was an unkind child. "Chinky" was the name she gave me, for my slightly smaller almond-shaped eyes—an outrageously racist term, even for that time and place. Up until that point I'd never really given my eyes much thought at all. And good grief, can you imagine the outrage if that xenophobic term was used today? The '80s and '90s weren't just a different time; in outback Australia, we were on a different planet—and let's face it, the hairstyles of the day can confirm that. Of course, after being christened "Chinky," I went a good two or three years in family and school photos with my eyes forced unnaturally wide, giving the impression of someone recently startled or under the influence of some kind of illicit substance (not a good look in hindsight).

My poor mother was perplexed to say the least. "Jane, try and look natural!" she'd holler at me, camera in hand, as I stood looking like I'd just been electrocuted. We were a family of shouters really. Learned behaviors indeed.

Sally found herself the recipient of universal karma in a rather more natural way. Despite mocking my unacceptably small eyes, Sally herself wasn't genetically blessed—at least not in the follicular department. You see, Sally was born with a head of hair consisting of small, tight curls that were challenging to manage at the best of times. To be fair, when long it was quite pretty. As white as salt, so light was the shade.

Now I will always wonder if a trainee hairdresser or Sally's mother was responsible for the following situation. Perhaps the heat got too much? I'll never know. But it was the summer, and we've all been known to make poor choices when the temperature rises. Well, I never did find out whose choice it was to give Sally an allover haircut that fateful day, but nevertheless, they did. Overnight she went from long, pretty hair to a one-inch buzz cut all over her head, giving poor Sally the appearance of white, old people pubic hair in entirely the wrong region. Tight, short, and curly in the extreme, I don't think I've ever seen a more unfortunate haircut. It was dreadful, and from that day forward, she was known as Pube Head. Suddenly someone at school had a bigger problem than I. I may have been Rowlf the Muppet, but mercifully the hair on my head wasn't ever, not once, compared to the hair found on one's nether regions.

Again, there was a God.

I feel it essential to stress that at sixteen, I found Amanda Wilson's widening derriere amusing; at forty-five, I do not. Nor would I laugh now at someone's unfortunate haircut. At that point in my life when I was bullied, my dark sense of humor relished these karmic events. Possessing far more kindness and compassion now in my mid-forties, I wish to make clear that I take no amusement in someone's weight struggles; after all, I've spent a lifetime being judged for mine. How unwittingly we become participants in our oppression, perpetuating these social norms. *Will it ever end?*

I'll never forget the time that I'd grown rapidly (mercifully up, not out, this time) and had nothing to wear for PE—that humiliating class in which we would all line up and wait to be picked by one of the popular team captains. And why did the teacher always play favorites? In any event, this day my humiliation was twofold: Not only was I one of the remaining few to be chosen for the cricket team (yes, really), I was also mocked for wearing an old brown and green tracksuit that my mother had given me. Someone creative pointed out that I looked much like a tree, and unfortunately, they were correct on this point. I did resemble a deciduous tree at the height of summer. I also recall being the only one who didn't find this funny.

scales

Shame is the intensely painful feeling or experience of believing that we are flawed and therefore unworthy of love and belonging.

—Brené Brown

"Oh look, it's fatty and skinny!" I close my eyes, and I'm twelve again, walking alongside a friend and into the schoolyard.

Asshole.

And I was by no means fat. That came later. I was solid, sturdy. My friend was leaner, lithe. More acceptable for the culture of the day. It was 1990 after all. The waif madness was all the fashion. Suddenly society demanded that women starve themselves into some Kate Moss contortion of bones and desire. Appetite be damned. Who needed food when we could starve ourselves and look like the anorexic models that graced the magazine covers of the day?

As a young child, food was neutral. Completely. I have to go a long way back, but there was a time. The smiling girl with her ponytails and ribbons had yet to discover the power of food as comfort in times of pain, an escape in times of overwhelm. She simply ate, enjoyed the meal, and then went about her day. *Just when did that all change?* I wondered. *Where did she go?*

I recall a math exercise in grade six. The teacher brought in scales. We were all lined up, all thirty of us in our green and white public-school uniforms, and we were weighed and measured, in full view of everyone. The numbers recorded on the chalkboard, the lesson evidently one of graphing, statistics. It was the late-1980s—this would never be allowed today. I still recall my heart thumping. I remember the fear.

I was on the tall side for my age, having begun that inevitable change from girl to woman a little early. To be clear, I wasn't in danger of being bowled over by a gust of wind anytime soon (carrying a few extra pounds by this stage). After all, I'd discovered baking. Sadly, on that unfortunate day in grade six, I also discovered shame. The petite girls in my class with their perfect hair, perfect families, and perfectly matching lunchboxes had numbers that fell below my own. Sometimes considerably. The boys chuckled; bullying was rife. "Teasing," we called it back then. Schools typically shrugged it off. Kids will be kids. We now know just how incredibly damaging this is. The beginnings of a decades-long war with my body and its sturdy frame. If only I had the perfect lunchbox, the lean limbs of the popular girl with her swimming pool and mother who was unfailingly at the gate at 3:00 p.m. for school pickup. This was not my experience. My mother wasn't at the gate with a smile and snacks. She was at work. Her full-time career put food on our table. My father did not.

Looking back, this experience highlights in stark relief the damage that can be caused when we focus upon a child's weight. A single number. And my number told me that I wasn't good enough; I was too much. Too heavy. Big-boned, my mother called me. Her intention wasn't to cause harm; she saw it as a fact. Of course, years later, as the weight went on and then off, much to everybody's surprise, I didn't have big bones at all. I have a perfectly lovely set of bones, and I'm grateful for them. What I had was decades of emotional eating hiding my frame—average-sized for five foot nine. Big bones I did not have. Quite the revelation really, and frankly, I think my mother is still surprised by the healthy frame that was unearthed when I finally made peace with my body.

In grade twelve, I recall a rather unfortunate foray into the world of diet pills. My dearest friend Kellie and I had (of course) decided that we both needed to lose some weight. It was 1995 after all, and at this point, the waif look was still everywhere. An entire generation of impressionable teenage girls received a very clear message: Thin was in. Actually, let's call it what it was: Emaciated. After all, I'm pretty sure some of those models died. They certainly looked close to death with their hollowed-out cheeks and vacant stares. Of course, some women are built this way, are indeed naturally slender. Kellie and I were not. To be fair, Kellie was a far closer approximation than I. Much to my chagrin, I was already sporting what my mother lovingly termed thunder thighs, and they were about as far away from the runway waif look as a person could get.

Anyway, back to the unfortunate day in question. Kellie and I, in our infinite wisdom, decided that the perfect adjunct to the diet pills was a walk. A solid plan, yes? What we didn't factor in was the rather enthusiastic (read: reckless) decision to take double the suggested dose. If one was effective, imagine what two could do for my thunder thighs!

We soon learned exactly what diet pills in the '90s did to a person's digestive system. They are, after all, loaded with caffeine (a known laxative) and Lord knows what else. We also failed to take into account the events of that morning. Now Kellie's mother Gloria—a practical and thrifty mother of five children—had an impressive grove of perfectly ripe stone fruit trees in her garden. It was the height of summer, and we ate like the gods, feasting on scrumptious apricots. Unfortunately, this excessive apricot consumption was timed just before the consumption of the diet pills and ensuing walk. We decided that a walk out of our small country town might be pleasant. To this day I have no idea why. We were both an inordinate distance from the nearest flushing toilet when the apricots, the diet pills, and the scorching Australian sun took effect. I don't recommend this course of action for rapid weight loss. Or any weight loss.

The diet pills went in the trash, and it was weeks before I could so much as look at Gloria's fruit trees that had once been a source of delight. I'm still not sure my stomach has forgiven me for this moment of madness.

Sadly, thirty years later I see that diet pills are still being peddled to impressionable teens, who are told via our toxic Instagram world that they, too, are not enough. Not thin enough, not airbrushed enough. Not impossibly perfect enough. Will this madness ever end? Yes, the body positive and body neutrality movements are gaining traction, but we still have a very long way to go. While the patriarchy continues to demand that women conform to unrealistic, often unattainable body shapes, eating disorders will continue to plague generation after generation of young people. I use "young people" instead of "girls," because an increasing number of boys are now accruing their own alarming statistics in addition to those who identify as nonbinary, as my eldest does.

Writing about this time in my life is proving difficult, which is exactly why my story must be told. If but one person benefits from reading my tale, then the vulnerability required to share this will be reward enough. I chose a career in counseling for this very reason: to help. From the depths of my soul, I feel the need to share these experiences. My wish is to help the millions of emotional eaters who were also told, often at a very young age, that they were not enough. Or perhaps too much. Too loud. Too big. Too opinionated. After all, good girls were quiet. Submissive. Demure. Agreeable. Slender.

To my maternal grandmother, I was everything a young lady shouldn't be. I was loud, opinionated, and—God forbid—educated in the public system with the great unwashed. This is a woman who was raised with servants, and suffice to say, my lack of private school education was entirely unacceptable. Ladies were finished properly at boarding school, where they were "turned out," as she was, with the ability to be demure and who the fuck knows what else. All I know is that my parents couldn't afford to send me to boarding school, and as a result, I was even more of a disappointment to my grandmother.

My saddest memory with her is a Christmas Eve. I was around thirteen. On the precipice of everything teenaged, my body was changing. My breasts, in hindsight, were lovely, and I was wearing a very pretty floral dress. As soon as we were alone, my grandmother took it upon herself to inform me that she didn't like the dress on me at all.

"It makes you look *fat.*"

Oh, how those words cut, spoken with unconcealed venom. My eyes stung with the tears of a vulnerable young girl who wanted nothing more or less than to be loved. That was never to be. Conceived out of wedlock, I was forever destined to be the bastard child of a working-class divorcé and my just-out-of-college mother. Quite the scandal in my grandmother's world. Rural Australia in 1977 was still exceedingly conservative, and nice girls from good families simply didn't fall pregnant to a thirty-year-old divorcé from the wrong side of town. So, she marched them down the aisle, and I attended the wedding—in utero.

The photo of the mothers of the bride and groom sitting in the pews could have been taken at a funeral—such was the nature of their expressions. And I have to wonder, what effect did that stress and negativity have on myself, a developing baby in the womb? After all, my mother briefly considered an abortion. Rather thankful that didn't happen. So, you see, I wasn't good enough, even before I was born. Perhaps on some level my soul was aware of this coming into the world.

dad

Forgiveness is just another name for freedom.

—Byron Katie

When we hit a child, we drastically increase the likelihood that they will use similar disciplinary measures with their own children. I don't remember what I'd done that day, but when I close my eyes and think about it, I'm five years old again. And this hurts every atom in my body to write. Perhaps because in writing this it's real again. I can hear my mother behind me, imploring my father to stop. My bottom bare, the welts from the belt red, angry, and burning, and I'm crying. I feel sick when I think that this was considered acceptable discipline in the early '80s. Acceptable for a father to take the belt from his pants, pull down my own, and proceed to belt my tiny body into submission. I'd been cheeky, had probably answered back—he snapped. Still doesn't make it okay, does it?

Ten years old in the front garden. Lord only knows what I'd done that time. It can't have been much as I don't recall. What I recall is the pain. His belt, on the back of my bare, tanned legs this time. And it burned like hell. I also learned that day what not to say to my father at the wrong time.

Defiant, I met his gaze with my own steely determination. "Didn't hurt," I lied.

I threw the words at him with as much attitude as my ten-year-old soul could muster, then I ran. Past the front lawn and out to the backyard, past the forklift and the overgrown lemon tree and the weeds that flourished beneath its wild limbs. I don't know how long I stayed away. Long enough to prevent another belting, I remember that much.

Looking back, there's no anger now, just a deep sadness. Sadness for the children who needed a better father. And sadness for the man who wasn't coping with fatherhood, who couldn't possibly cope with the monumental responsibility he'd assumed. And sadness for the woman who should have walked away far sooner than she did.

I don't want pity. Mine is not a tale of horrific abuse, despite these isolated and intermittent moments. Having said that, I do recall another unfortunate form of discipline. There's just no end to the pain one human can inflict upon another when they try, is there?

Family road trips. At least five or six hours to get anywhere, from one dot on the map to another. Backseat arguing was a constant between my sister Laura and me. After all, there really wasn't much else to do: I'd read. We'd pass the odd kangaroo, a few emus (quite possibly the stupidest bird on the planet). And we'd bicker. My father, never one to have been blessed with patience, would snap—he was prone to this, really. Pinching me in anger, he'd reach his hands from the front passenger seat around the back to my waiting legs, bare due to the endless summer heat. And it bloody hurt.

And why was Mum always driving? Dad would sleep. Why? So many questions.

Was it any wonder that food became so very comforting? You see, food didn't pinch me from the back seat.

They say there's a black sheep in every family, and mine was no exception. Having said that, my father did have a few redeeming qualities. We all possess darkness and light within, and my father frequently demonstrated both—he was nothing if not inconsistent.

"Jane, the world is divided into two types of people!" he'd tell me. "There are people who are kind to animals, and there are people who are cruel."

Very astute.

My father, being in the kind camp, would return home from Lord knows where on a regular basis with some stray animal or another. A kitten in his top pocket, an unwanted dog in the back seat of the car. My mother drew the line at the baby goat. After all, that thing stank to high heaven. I don't know if you've ever been up close to a goat, but they have a rather pungent aroma that neither myself nor my mother could abide.

"Michael, get rid of it," she demanded. "Today."

Jan put her foot down, and the goat was gone by dinnertime.

hijinks

As soon as I saw you, I knew an
adventure was going to happen.

—Winnie the Pooh

The father I wanted lived next door. Jack Edwards was everything my father wasn't. He called me Janey, and in my eyes, he was the perfect dad. His warm eyes smiled at my antics, he laughed at my fearless energy and enthusiasm, and most importantly, he always made me feel loved.

Recently I received a phone call. I immediately sensed the foreboding nature of the conversation, despite the distance.

"Jane, Jack Edwards has died." The sadness in my mother's voice on the phone was palpable. Shock flooded my body, and for the first time in my life, I felt true grief for someone who had crossed over, from this world into the next. And I cried.

Why is it that the good are taken too early? One month into retirement, and Jack was diagnosed with MND. He declined rapidly, and six months later he was gone. Just like that, leaving a wonderful woman and two grown sons behind. Jack was the kind of rare man that our world dearly needs more of. Eyes full of laughter and kindness, he worked hard to provide for his family. Back and forth to the silver, lead, and zinc mine. Decades of shift work. An honest life.

On the weekends he'd renovate. Constantly improving the family home, I'd chat with him over the old, corrugated iron fence that separated his idyllic backyard from my own rambling quarters. Sometimes I'd assist him, eager to be helpful and always happy in his presence.

"Jane, you'd better be getting home now for dinner. It's getting dark out," he'd tell me gently. But I didn't want to go home. Back to the messy, disorganised house? No, thank you. I wanted to stay right where I was.

"Jane, I swear some mornings it's like you're underneath our bed shouting!" Helen, Jack's beautiful widow, told me more than once, laughing. And I was loud. You see, I had to shout to be heard in my childhood home. It was the only way. Less than ideal, our kitchen had the misfortune to be placed directly opposite Jack and Helen's bedroom window, with the corrugated fence doing naught to provide a sound barrier. After all, we could all hear the teenaged boy playing his drums two doors down. How Helen and Jack tolerated the ruckus for so long I will never know.

My baking also disturbed their peace. After school I'd bake my own snacks. There was little guidance. My father was in his own world (God knows where), and my mother was busy working. Always busy. So, I'd cook up a storm. I recall the chocolate cake, the chocolate coconut slice, the cheesecake set with lemon juice in the fridge, and all manner of biscuits. It was relaxing, really. The problem was in the consumption. Just no moderation. Of course, for my long-suffering neighbors, this was less than ideal for other reasons. After all, I was in the kitchen where they could hear a pin drop, hollering at a volume that could wake the dead, and continuing to disturb poor Helen, usually busy with housework (I was in constant awe of her pristine home).

I think about Jack Edwards often. I like to imagine that my daily antics with my children would amuse him, as it's my turn now at this madness we call parenthood. After all, if there's a world beyond this one, and if Jack is inhabiting it, then he has time to spare. Eternity isn't short on time. And I know he'd be checking up on me occasionally. I only hope I can make him proud of the too-loud girl who lived next door.

Fun fact! One town in Australia holds the unfortunate record for having the most obese number of citizens per capita in the entire country. Quite the sobering statistic, and yes, you guessed it! Broken Hill. This unfortunate community also holds the distinction of having many of its citizens possess dangerously high levels of lead in their bloodstreams. You see, the home of my formative years was also home to the largest silver, lead, and zinc deposit the world had ever seen. One can only imagine just how much lead dust blanketed the community after 150 years of mining activity. The town grew around the accumulating waste dumps of dirt that stood mere blocks away from the main shopping and residential districts. It was unfortunate that no one had the foresight to place the community just a little farther away from the mine site. Of course, in 1883, no one had any clue as to the dangers that lead posed.

Judging from the behaviors of some of my classmates, I saw firsthand the consequences of lead exposure. If I'm not painting some kind of idyllic oasis in the desert, it's for good reason. Broken Hill was quite the opposite. To this day I remain grateful to have escaped at eighteen—I imagine that was quite enough lead exposure for one lifetime.

Kellie and I certainly found ways to pass the time while we awaited our respective departures. Jane Hijinx and Kellie Tomfoolery were our code names. We essentially did rather silly things periodically and amused ourselves with alter egos. Such was the nature of small-town life: Amusing oneself was the only entertainment. Without the plethora of modern tech that our children now devour to pass the time, we had to make our own fun, and I'm pleased to report that we did. There was such innocence to those days. And a safety. Bullying was hurtful, no question, but it blessedly ended with the school bell. No social media and the 24-7 cyberbullying of today that our children contend with. Mercifully we were blessed with a childhood devoid of this (and a bloody good thing in hindsight, given that we all had to endure the lead exposure. Ninety-nine problems indeed).

The corner store was a curious establishment due to the peculiarities of its proprietor, Richard—a long-term Broken Hill resident. It's likely that he, too, was affected by a lifetime of lead dust, the poor fellow. Being in close proximity to both my crazy home and Kellie's busy abode, we'd often head over there for the forty-cent ice creams or two-cent milk lollies. How I never broke a tooth on one remains a mystery. Sweet, hard, and gooey, it took a sturdy jaw to soften and eventually swallow these artificial vanilla treats. I always did succeed— never one to quit!

There was but one riddle we could never solve: Whenever we would enter the store, Richard would race to the back of the store and simply disappear for some time. Did he suffer from anthropophobia—a fear of people? Did he have hidden cameras with which he'd spy on patrons? So of course, it became a game. We'd repeatedly enter, and the same predictable behavior of the owner would follow, Pavlovian-dog style. Did he not want to take our money? He would eventually return to the front of the store to serve us, but I recall that he never did meet our inquisitive gaze. I concluded that he was likely just as mad as a cut snake, another victim of lead poisoning, the poor bastard.

There was sometimes a third participant in our shenanigans: Dion, my requisite gay friend (and yes, of course he has fabulous style—stereotypes exist for a reason, after all). Well, Dion had the misfortune of driving his parent's old Charger after gaining his driver's license. The thing was, the car was so old and in such a state of disrepair, that neither the speedometer nor the seatbelts worked. Kellie and I essentially took our lives into our own hands every time we jumped in for a joyride, which was quite often. There was precious little to do otherwise in this uninspiring town. I recall the wind in our hair as we'd fly over the overpass connecting south to north Broken Hill, having absolutely no idea how fast we were traveling, past the mountainous waste piles of lead-filled dirt. If our disheveled hair was any indication, it was excessive and wildly unsafe.

My car wasn't much better. It cost my father $500 and looked like it cost less. Driven by a little old lady to church for thirty years before the sale, it actually ran pretty well. It was also blessed with license plates that began with QRG, looking close enough to ORG to be christened the Org-Mobile. Filthy jokes flowed like my wild hair in Dion's car. It eventually died years later when, as a poor university student, I had the brilliant idea to change the oil myself. The manual said the oil capacity was 1.7 liters, so that's exactly what I added. Now, if you're reading this and have any basic automotive knowledge, you will know what comes next. I turned the engine on, feeling quite proud of my efforts. Well, the car was immediately engulfed in dark grey smoke. To any unfortunate passerby in the neighborhood, it looked like something was seriously ablaze. And much like the music, that was the day the Org-Mobile died.

Friday nights required creativity, and we seemed to possess just enough resourcefulness to avoid the binge-drinking benders of our peers. Instead, we'd take my parents old '70s Mercedes sedan, which must have weighed several tons, and in the dark, we'd drive to the top of the largest nonbroken hill we could find. Getting to the top, I had the genius idea to throw the car into neutral and barrel down this very steep hill, gaining speed rapidly and then braking at the very last second. The town of our youth didn't have an amusement park—it didn't need one. We made our own! Looking back, it's a wonder we never ended up in the parlour of the poor elderly couple that lived across the street, careening through their living room. Or dead. How we all survived our collective childhoods in Broken Hill is still beyond me.

vomit

Be kind, for everyone that you meet is fighting a battle that you know nothing about.

—Wendy Mass

I was about nineteen when I first vomited. Anxiety.

Of course, I didn't know at the time that this was anxiety. I thought perhaps I'd eaten something bad. I remember it well. I was on a Greyhound bus, and let's face it, the smell alone on those unfortunate modes of transportation is enough to make anyone hurl. The recycled AC—that faint, stale scent that you can't quite pinpoint. You just know that there's likely a story behind it. Possibly another anxious vomiter, the poor bastard.

Fortunately, I managed to contain the contents of my stomach for the duration of my eight-hour ordeal en route to a family reunion. My grandmother would be in attendance—hence my apprehension. It was dark out. I remember the stars overhead and my mother's backyard, the warm breeze, and my retching. I vomited until the bile came up, and I collapsed, at that point somewhat dehydrated, I'm sure. I hadn't been able to keep water down in hours.

The next morning, I started eating. No doubt physically hungry this time, yet once again food made a wonderful substitute for love. Food didn't criticize. Blessedly devoid of judgment, it never made me feel less than. Hungry for acceptance, and my poor stomach growling after my anxiety-vomiting bender, I ate.

Looking back, it saddens me to think of the effect that my grandmother's distain for my existence had on my self-esteem. Criticism at every turn. The sun shined from the other grandchildren; they could do no wrong. Not an uncommon story in many extended families, yet a sad one just the same. If only the adults in a child's precious, vulnerable childhood were aware of even a fraction of the power of their words and actions. Aware of the damage they inflict. Countless clients walk through my office door with raw emotional wounds, the result of scars born in childhoods lacking in love, abundant in dysfunction and pain.

Mother worked tirelessly to pay the bills, living paycheck to paycheck. She always ensured we had opportunities, but we knew very well that there was never a surplus. Golf was Jan's escape. It still is, only now she's escaping for different reasons.

My father had a great many problems, and one of them was running up bills that he simply couldn't afford to pay. Long distance phone calls at that time weren't cheap. To this day I still don't know who he was phoning, but I remember all too well the humiliation at netball practice, when Sophie asked me, "Jane, why is your phone line disconnected? Didn't your parents pay the bill?" All seven teammates turned to stare, some curious. Not one look of pity, but perhaps that was for the best. No one wants pity. The shame and humiliation ran deep. I knew damn well that my mother was faced with a $1000-plus bill that she couldn't cover.

This situation was repeated several times throughout my childhood. Once we even had the electricity cut off, albeit briefly. To a teenager who wanted so badly to have a normal family, I was continually mortified by mine. Food was a precious comfort at these times. An escape from the shame.

"You should leave him," I'd tell my mother. Infrequently at first, and then regularly. She was so clearly unhappy, biding her time. Buy why? I realize that for many people, my mother being one of them, change is frightening. Unwelcome. Better the devil you know. Ironically, change is the only constant in life. Well, that and death, but let's not dwell on that. After all, I have a book to write. I don't have time to die.

The anxiety-induced vomiting continued throughout much of my twenties. Sadly, not enough to reduce my waistline, but enough to raise an alarm from my mother and new husband Brian. I'd married young, you see, rushing into the institution soon after university graduation—barely out of my childhood and far too young to have any idea of the momentous commitment that I was making.

One woman who likely knew exactly what I was barreling into was Australian social activist, Irina Dunn. Her immortal words truer today than ever before: "A woman needs a man like a fish needs a bicycle."

How I love that an Aussie coined this phrase! At the age of forty-five, I agree wholeheartedly; at twenty-five, I didn't. Why did I need a man? Who taught me this? We don't have to look very far to see that the small patriarchal town of my youth was implicit in this deception.

Up until the late 1970s in Broken Hill, a woman was expected to give up her job upon marriage, making the position available for an unwed girl. This was an unspoken (and illegal) but enforced local rule. A staunch union town, there was no argument. How this archaic practice survived so long I will never know. It was simply never a question one asked. I grew up with the understanding that I would marry and raise a family. I don't ever recall questioning the process. It seemed like the logical next step after completing my education. Boy and girl meet at university, date, move in together, buy joint appliances, etc. Engagement at twenty-three. Marriage followed at twenty-four, pregnant at twenty-five, baby at twenty-six. My third at thirty.

And why did I rush into marriage at such a young age? We don't have to look far to see the glaring daddy issues. Of course, I was bound to marry the first responsible man I met. He was the very opposite of my father and for that reason alone close to perfect in my eyes. When you are born to a man incapable of the responsibilities of marriage and father-hood, any reliable, steady man is a revelation—something to hold on to, and tightly.

I was also driven by a determination not to make the same mistakes my mother did. Laura and I witnessed her struggles firsthand. Brian equaled security and safety, two things my mother's union lacked in spades. Did I ignore signs that we weren't entirely compatible? Of course I did! Insecure and craving the consistency and safety of a steady, reliable boyfriend, not once did I question our trajectory. And so, we dove headfirst into responsibilities, far too young.

"Brian, I really don't feel good. My head hurts. I need to throw up. I'm so sorry." I force the words out, not wanting any communication. Craving the darkness. Apologizing.

Always apologizing.

"Can I get you anything?"

"No thank you, I just need rest."

Lying down, I look up at the cassette-tape-era blue of the walls in Brian's childhood bedroom. Who chose this dreadful shade of blue? And why?! Failing to distract myself, I hear my mother-in-law, Cheryl, in the hallway.

"Is it food poisoning? Perhaps she picked up a bug on the flight. Oh dear. Well, I hope we don't catch it!" Cheryl really didn't sound thrilled about the whole thing. Unbeknownst to her, I was well aware that my stomach-in-knots situation was driven by my anxiety disorder. There was a BBQ that day, in honor of our arrival, complete with extended friends and family. Now on an anxiety rating scale from one to ten, this type of event would send me careening up to about a twenty. I don't even recognize this anxious girl anymore. Who was she, and how could potential judgment from her in-laws send her spiraling into such a state that she had to take to bed?

In hindsight, this was my body's way of saying, *I'm done. I don't want to be here. I need a break.* It was my stop-the-world-I-want-to-get-off moment. And so, I did. I threw up later that afternoon, until there was nothing left to bring up. The contents of my poor, weary stomach completely empty. The bile acidic, burning my esophagus as I wretched. And then I'd sleep, welcoming the darkness.

Kellie recalls another time, after another in-law visit. The scene was her driveway. An eleven-hour road trip ahead of us, all three children young, and I was ill. Her husband still laughs, years later.

"Do you remember the time you threw up in the bushes, Jane? In the front yard?!" Kellie asks.

"Yes, yes I do." All too well. Tears streaming down my face, my whole body just wanting to shut down and sleep for a good twelve hours in a dark room. But I couldn't. "God, that was awful." Such was the stress around visiting my in-laws.

You see, I just never felt quite good enough. Not slim enough. Not demure enough. And my father was a constant source of embarrassment.

"How is your father, Jane? Do you hear from him much?" Cheryl would ask.

"No, no I don't. Not often." He'd make promises back then, never following through. I learned long ago to take them with a grain of salt. Sadly, my younger sister would believe them, forever hopeful, forever disappointed. She'd inevitably find herself crushed. Shakespeare was right: Expectations are indeed the root of all heartache.

My father's intentions were good. I know he loved us all. I've never doubted this. He also wanted to be able to provide for us financially, he just never seemed to be able to get it all together. I do believe that our parents all truly do the best they can, with the knowledge and capacity that they have at the time. Sadly, my father fell woefully short in his capacity to parent. And as my high school geography teacher would share with me years before, "The road to hell is paved with good intentions, Jane!"

I couldn't help but agree.

inappropriate

If you can't say anything nice,
then don't say anything at all.

—Aesop

"**H**ello, Big Girl!"
This unfortunate greeting came from one of my mother-in-law's dearest friends. We had just flown in, two small children in tow at this time. I was carrying not only the baby weight of two back-to-back pregnancies, but also the weight of my emotional eating disorder. And the words stung. Why is it that thin people feel the need to tell us when we've gained weight? Do they actually think that we don't know? Did Elaine think that I was somehow unaware of the excess flesh that I so despised? The pants in a bigger size? Did she think I didn't own a full-length mirror? (I did.)

Overweight people don't need thinly veiled insults from the slim. They need kindness and compassion. Did Elaine think that this greeting would somehow motivate me to suddenly head out for a quick 10 km run? *My God, thank you! I had no idea that I'd recently gained fifty pounds. Bless you for pointing that out!*

Frankly, I don't think I even owned workout gear at this point in my life. Did I?

Too tired from the responsibilities I shouldered to exercise or even care much about fitness at this stage. Exhausted by the demands of full-time motherhood and my eldest, who was showing signs of autism. Those were the days of survival. Childcare and sleep. Two priorities. Everything else seemed superfluous. Including a 10 km run. Well intentioned, shaming comments do nothing to help. It doesn't work like that. Fuckwits.

And what did I do that day? I ate, snacking and grazing my way through the afternoon in an attempt to avoid the hurt and humiliation, numbing my feelings with whatever my mother-in-law had in her kitchen (another experience altogether. . . . Nothing if not frugal, Cheryl would hold onto food well past expiration dates). Deeply entrenched behaviors from my childhood, continually reinforced. I was on autopilot, at this point unaware of the root of my self-destructive patterns. That awareness would come later.

I recall possibly the most horrifying realization of my altered postbaby form. We'd just had a roll of film developed. Yes, these were still the days of a twenty-four-exposure roll of film. No endless snapping of iPhone selfies to capture the perfect shot. Oh no. You had twenty-four chances, and good luck to you!

Well, evidently, we failed. My mother had taken a few new baby pics, and one at a distance. I recall ripping open the paper, eager to see how the film turned out.

"What is *that*?!" I exclaimed with disdain. I thought we'd accidently taken a photo of a random, unfashionably dressed, overweight person.

And then it hit me.

Oh fuck.

That frumpy, overweight person was me.

Standing at a distance next to the pram, unaware that the photo was taken at all. Well God help me if that wasn't a wake-up call. I was mortified. Who knew I'd actually left the house in that state?!

Looking back, I realize that I was a new mother, breast-feeding and sleep deprived—I couldn't have cared less what I was wearing at that point. If only I'd offered myself compassion, but I was years away from learning that lesson. And I was hungry. I was nursing a newborn with a voracious appetite. One of the few times in my life that I felt physical hunger, as my body demanded nutrition to fuel my baby's growth. Being iron deficient didn't help either, nor did my unawareness of this. The sugar cravings were out of control. Simple carbs for energy: toast with Vegemite or apricot jam and butter. What my body actually needed was more protein. Healthy carbs. And sleep. And I also needed to burn that God-awful photo, which I think I did years later. Or perhaps it was shredded? I'm not sure. It doesn't matter. That image is burned into my brain.

Every person who has recovered from disordered eating has those photos. The ones that fill us with shame, horror, and in time, sadness. Then eventually acceptance. Acceptance of a time in my life when I was struggling. In need of help. We were thousands of miles away from extended family and friends. Marriage to a mining engineer meant remote locations, small towns, and long, dull car rides to get just about anywhere, including the seven-hour car ride to the hospital where I was to give birth to my son, thirty years after my own birth in that same small-town hospital. Deniliquin.

Looking into the pram, Brian's colleague, Angela, exclaimed, "Oh, he's beautiful!"

"I didn't even know you were pregnant! Congratulations!"

"Well, yes, yes, I was. For the last nine months actually . . ."

The hurt hidden behind humor, always hidden. A common technique.

"I had no idea!" Angela repeated, quite without thought. To be fair, she looked slightly uncomfortable after realizing her faux pas. Having just run into her, I was rather alarmed to learn that apparently over the last nine months, I appeared to the general public not to be pregnant with my third child, but steadily gaining weight. Did this small community just think I was eating too many pies?!

Apparently yes. Good Lord.

Of all the things you don't say to a woman with a newborn, I'm pretty sure this is at the top of the list. Clearly, she just thought I was getting fatter! I was mortified, but in typical Jane style, I hid it all rather well behind my smile.

"That's just so rude," was Kellie's take on the situation. "Seriously, even if you think that, you don't say it."

Agreed.

"And you *did* look pregnant!" she added.

Bless Kellie and her supportive heart.

In reality, I probably did look much like a "before" contestant on *The Biggest Loser*. And I felt like crap. Some women bounce back from multiple pregnancies with washboard stomachs. I still don't know how, and clearly this was not my experience. Mine was vastly different.

"I had no idea that women got so big when they were pregnant!" commented another friend and colleague of my husband's.

"Yes, well, I am about to have a baby, Ryan."

Why is it that people feel the need to say such wildly inappropriate things to pregnant women? Where the fuck is their filter? There's something curious about pregnancy, something that seems to allow people to lose all sense of decency. Not only did my changing form now belong to the baby growing inside me, it apparently also belonged to every fucker on the planet who felt that they had the right to comment, appraise, and even touch my growing stomach. It was all very unsettling really.

"Wow! You look like you're having twins!"

Another day. Another inappropriate comment.

Even if I did look to be carrying more than one baby, did the young girl at the greengrocers think that this was the best thing to share that day? Nine months pregnant and glowing from the sweat of our January heat, I was not amused. As always, I hid it with a smile.

"No, no, there's just one in here. Well, according to the ultrasound anyway!"

Idiot.

I ate for England. Zero morning sickness meant immediate weight gain. And why is it that, at the one time in my life that I was supposed to throw up, I couldn't?!

"Jane! You've gotten so fat!" Ahh, the words of my grandmother-in-law. What was it with me and grandmothers? Had I killed one in a former life? I was certainly paying for it in this one. Geez.

And why is it that when someone reaches their eighth decade, they suddenly feel the need to say exactly what they're thinking? Zero filter. Have they earned that right by virtue of not dying? I would argue no.

Another day, another smile to hide the hurt. Wandering past a man-made lake, the fresh, heady scent of the mowed lawn at the local gardens pleasantly saturated my excessive frame. Later, wandering the local stores, we passed a rack of bikinis on sale.

I couldn't believe that she said the following to me next either, but she did. And it stung. My mother-in-law and grandmother-in-law were visiting. Again. I was eight months pregnant.

"Well, you won't be wearing these, Jane!" My grand-mother-in-law chuckled.

"No, no, I won't."

She really did have an incredible grasp of the obvious.

"Oh, Mum. Really?!" my mother-in-law replied. Even she objected to that comment.

Now I'll admit that in that moment, I had some rather unkind thoughts about the elderly lady before me who was clearly lacking a filter. And one month later she was dead. I'd like to stress here from a massive stroke, not of my own doing. Nevertheless, my friends like to joke that I'm probably the last person on Earth that you want to piss off. Just to be safe.

the fridge

The road of excess leads to the palace of wisdom.

—William Blake

"**J**ane, there won't be any left for dinner at this rate!"

Ahh . . . the critical voice of my mother-in-law. I should note that the food in question was a pasta salad I'd prepared as a side to have on the dinner table.

"But I'm starving!" I exclaimed as I helped myself to the delicious tomato, basil, and feta in my favorite blue salad bowl. Now starving was likely a stretch, but I was hungry that day. Nursing my newborn, chasing my one-year-old and in-law houseguests to boot. It's a wonder I was reaching for salad at all. Let's just all take a moment to be thankful for the fact that I didn't develop a drinking problem around this time. Thinly veiled criticisms were a regular occurrence back then.

"You don't need butter on that sandwich, Jane!" I looked up, taken aback by the inappropriate statement. Now the wild irony here is that my mother-in-law isn't the smallest woman herself, having gained considerable weight during menopause. But that didn't stop her from dishing out her own dietary advice to her daughter-in-law. Oh no! That advice flowed like water down the creek after an outback thunderstorm.

"Hmm, I wonder where all of that went?" inquired Cheryl during breakfast. The remains of the banana caramel pie, found one morning in the refrigerator. Shame flooded my body, much like the sugar flooded my bloodstream that morning at 2:00 a.m. To be fair, I'd been awake and nursing. I knew exactly where it went. And so did Cheryl. Highlighting the obvious was hardly necessary. My escape was the kitchen. Exhausted, overwhelmed, and the last thing I'd wanted was houseguests—of any type. Hadn't somebody told them that houseguests, like chicken, went bad after three days? Clearly not. They stayed three weeks. And I coped with the extra demands the only way I knew how. I ate. Because the thing is, banana caramel pie didn't judge me. It didn't demand anything. There was no criticism. And it was delicious—I'd made it from scratch, after all. Like an alcoholic at a bar, resistance was futile.

Let's face it: If you're awake at 2:00 a.m. and houseguests are asleep, there's a freedom in being able to enjoy a few moments of solitude in one's own home. Not to mention, bloody well eat in peace without the judgment of said houseguests. Seriously. My 2:00 a.m. escape was chocolate, caramel, biscuits, banana, real cream. If there's a more perfect combination of ingredients for a pie, I'm yet to find it (and please feel free to email me the recipe. Ditto any potential FF nominees. Please don't hesitate to reach out via email with the tale of madness . . .).

Of course, I'd baked this pie as a treat. A celebration of the grandparents' arrival. In reality, I baked this because I wanted to, because I knew at 2:00 a.m. that this would be the only thing that I would want as I stumbled into the kitchen, hungry and exhausted from the demands of a new baby. As anyone with a newborn and a challenging one-year-old can attest, this is a rather difficult time. Add in-law houseguests to the mix for three weeks and I defy anyone not to comfort eat. Sadly, my comfort eating was out of control. Elastic waistbands were my friend.

Now when I say challenging one-year-old, this is no exaggeration. My eldest was exhibiting autistic traits even at this early age. How no one identified these until age seventeen, I will never know. One day a specialist mercifully pieced this puzzle together. A collective "aha!" moment. It suddenly all made sense. You see, Cerulean, at age one, was prone to overreacting. Well naturally we thought the poor kid was just prone to dramatics. As a neurodivergent child, this reaction was entirely predictable and understandable for a child with Autism Spectrum Disorder (ASD).

Cerulean's name has been changed throughout for privacy, and they have requested that this particular moniker be used throughout this book (they/them pronouns). I'm far too old-school to give any of my kids a hippie name, being something of a traditionalist when it comes to naming one's offspring. I've never understood why some people feel the need to burden their future heirs with names that are difficult to spell, difficult to pronounce, or simply bizarre. Do they not think, even for a second, that this poor child must carry the name for life? Or at least until the age of majority when they can mercifully change it, if they so wish, to something a little easier to write on forms. The mind boggles.

You see, as a child, I mistakenly believed that all rich people are intelligent. How wrong I was! Of course, I very quickly learned as an adult, particularly in the case of inherited wealth and some celebrities, that many rich people are idiots. Quite the revelation. And we only have to look at some of the names of their children to confirm this theory: Jermajesty, Audio Science, Pilot Inspektor, Slash. WTF? God help us all (and them).

As a child I felt vastly inferior around the elite. Completely. After all, my parents couldn't always pay the bills. Mine was not a privileged upbringing. And so I'd eat, food yet again that reliable escape, my safe space. Comfortable until my pants were anything but. And ironically, the more weight I gained, the less confident I felt around anyone, wealthy or otherwise. But I do remain grateful for my given names: Jane Louise. Not even remotely offensive, and I've always secretly liked my name. But I digress. Again. Back to the tale of my eldest.

"No, honey, not now."

Cerulean wanted something, I can't remember what, but the answer was a regretful "No!" Now I know both as a parent, and someone with a decent amount of life experience, that responding with no to an eighteen-month-old will elicit a wide range of reactions from the child in question. When my second child Emily heard no at age one, she may have frowned or quietly protested, but quickly accepted the answer with all the grace and calm of a Buddhist monk. My firstborn, on the other hand, refused to accept a negative response. Banging their head repeatedly on my mother's honey-stained wooden floorboards, they screamed. At length. I have to say, their passion, frustration, and persistence was impressive. As were the marks left on my poor child's forehead.

Parenthood really isn't for the faint of heart. I'm convinced that if any new parent knew what was to come, the human race would shrink in size within a generation or two. My dear Kellie puts it best: "Jane, if someone had told me as a teenager that at age forty, I'd have no money, more worries, less energy, and screaming teenagers who actively hate me, I'd have never grown up. Why would anybody choose this?!"

Indeed.

Goodness knows it wasn't Cerulean's fault that a diagnosis wasn't made yet.

"Strong willed."

"Difficult."

"Headstrong."

Observers regularly assumed that, because I had a disobedient child, I was somehow deficient in parenting skills. Judgment was rife. As if it wasn't enough that I felt judged by my mother-in-law and most of the general public for being overweight, I was also now being judged as a parent. A mother lacking effective discipline! When will we all stop judging each other and begin extending compassion and kindness?! Today if I see a mother and child struggling, my heart aches for both of them. It's all I can do not to offer help, as that's not always appropriate either. Motherhood is the toughest job on the planet, and anyone who says otherwise is delusional.

"Jaaaane! Brian's on the phone!" Jan shouted from the kitchen. (This really is a family trait)

"Thanks."

Laughing, she handed me the brick-like wall phone, still attached by its bland beige coil to the kitchen wall.

"What's so funny?" I inquired.

"Brian said the fridge has frozen over! I guess you're not there to open and close the door all day! It got too cold!"

Mother was amused. When her laughter subsided, she expressed her understandable concern. (To be clear, she was mostly amused.)

Good grief. I was less so. Mind you, I did think that perhaps it was time for a new refrigerator. Shouldn't this necessary household appliance be better at regulating temperature? Evidently ours did not. And did I really open the fridge door all day? Apparently. Visiting my mother at the time provided brief respite, and rare assistance with the children. You see, we never lived anywhere near extended family, ever. My children never went to daycare. Why would they? I was a stay-at-home mum. I was adamant about wanting to raise my own children. The problem was that I never had a break. Ever. Mine was truly a 24-7-365 situation, and it took a massive toll. My mental health suffered (although I was yet to recognize this), and my physical health followed suit.

My first break was four-year-old preschool. Cerulean screamed blue murder (like only my children can). Driving out of the carpark, I could still hear their screams. "*Mummmmmmmmmyyyyyyyyyyyy!*"

Dark glasses, crying, I forced myself to drive away. Hot, wet tears soaked my face and splashed onto my clothing. The preschool teacher had to lock the door. Turns out my kid was a runner. Tough love was what I'd been taught, and I reasoned that separation anxiety wasn't going to be helped if I remained or took them home. Multiply this by three: Three first days of preschool. Three days of screaming (theirs). Three days of crying (everyone's).

Food continued to be my refuge. Cheesecake slices were only two-thirds of the size they should have been. Only I knew why. Escaping the demands of the day, childcare, the floors, the dishwasher that needed packing for the umpteenth time, I'd wander into the kitchen multiple times a day, each time slicing off one delicious small slither of white chocolate cheesecake, one slice after another. (It's still delectable, by the way, just now something that I'd make once a decade, such is its power.) There was no restraint, but all the while there was no real hunger either. How could I feel hunger, grazing on cheesecake throughout the day? My escape from reality.

"Oh, I have to get that recipe!" exclaimed Beth. "The pieces are very small . . ." She was perplexed, commenting.

"Yes, I make them small as it's very rich," I told my playgroup friends. Only I knew the truth: They were small because I'd eaten a good third of each piece the day before. My dysfunctional eating was as creative as it was unhealthy.

Disordered eating, I know you well! (And I really did have a problem with cheesecake.)

Why didn't I just allow myself one full piece, sitting down at the table to enjoy it? Because I wasn't supposed to eat it. I was supposed to be a on a diet. I couldn't eat a cheesecake slice! Did I really think that the calories didn't count if I ate standing up? The size of my waistline said otherwise, telling a different story (turns out they did count).

No, to sit and eat would be to acknowledge that I was allowed to eat a piece, a full piece, and I couldn't let myself do that. Ahh, shame . . . my constant companion.

The sugar addiction began in my early teens, well before most of us knew the dangers of sugar. Back then dietary fat was the enemy. Everything was upside down, and my body certainly didn't respond well to the low-fat dogma of the day. (Did anybody's?!) Unless you've been living under a rock for the last few decades, you also know of the highly addictive nature of sugar. After all, the same areas of the brain that light up when an addict uses cocaine also light up when we ingest sugar. Is it any wonder it felt so good for so long? After all,

I wasn't ingesting illegal drugs; I didn't need to. I had a legal drug at my fingertips . . . in the kitchen! For some people their addiction is alcohol, cocaine, or sex—their escape from reality. Mine was food.

After giving birth to Alexander, I had one of those unfortunate moments that's seared into my brain, the memory forever vivid in Technicolor. The scene was the small-town, country hospital maternity ward. And it went like this: One of the midwives wandered over, back on duty after a shift change.

"Are you still going?!" she asked me, thinking that I'm still in labor.

The other midwife looked at her in horror, a silent conversation taking place before my eyes. "She had a baby boy!" exclaimed the other.

"Oh!"

With no idea what else to say, she went silent. Probably for the best at this point.

I stood there, equal parts fatigue and horror, and somehow also beyond caring. But it still hit home. She thought I was wandering the halls of the maternity ward, yet to give birth.

Fuck me.

"No, no, I'm not, but thank you for asking!" was what I said. Now what I wanted to say was, "Oh my God, do I actually still look pregnant?!"

There I was, in the small kitchen that this rural hospital provided for new mothers. Many are nursing and haven't eaten for a day or more during labor. I have to wonder, perhaps the kitchen is provided as hospitals know that the precooked food that they provide is complete shit? Equivalent perhaps to economy airline food.

So anyway, there I was, making two of my old trusty favorites, a piece of Vegemite toast and mug of hot Milo, when I'm informed of the fact that I still look pregnant. Wonderful. And yes, this was one of those defining moments that motivated me to make permanent healthy changes in my life that I've maintained for a good fifteen years.

washrooms

Always go to the bathroom when you have a chance.

—King George V

"Excuse me, ahh, it seems that your child has had an accident on the floor."

I looked down, and indeed she had. Beneath us there was a flood of biblical proportions, no small feat given that we were living in a semiarid desert.

"Oh my God. Oh dear. It's okay, honey." You see, my eldest had something of an issue with bathrooms. Washrooms. Public facilities. In Australia we simply say, "I'm going to the toilet," but I learned quickly that the word toilet is considered a little crass over here in North America. So, let's say bathroom.

So, there we were, my two- and four-year-olds in tow, matching dresses and ribbons. The whole nine yards. I'm eight months pregnant with my son (and evidently looking fat not pregnant), trying to post a parcel to Lord knows where. That's irrelevant to the story. What is relevant is the look on the young man's face when I shared the news of the newly formed lake of urine in the middle of the post office. It would have been impressive if it wasn't at that very moment soaking into the faded, worn carpet beneath us.

49

"Excuse me, do you have a mop? Some towels?" I enquire, attempting a smile.

"Ahh . . ." He had nothing. Was he in shock? Did he not grow up with younger siblings?

"Some paper towels? I have my hands full, you see. I'm so very, very sorry!" I'm talking fast at this point, after all, I was also standing in urine. The postal worker was as still as a statue, Harry Potter like—the poor man was petrified. The man behind me was aghast, and at this point trying to find dry land and some paper towel of his own to dry his loafers.

Is it any wonder that I was a comfort eater?! Of course, if someone belonging to the medical profession had figured out that my kid was on the spectrum at age four, and not seventeen, this would have made the intervening years slightly easier. After all, when you have a kid screaming for thirty minutes at the top of their lungs in public, being able to tell a passerby that your child is autistic does bring a measure of understanding. In my case people just assumed that I had a "problem kid" and was probably "not using suitable discipline within the home." (The opinion of one older woman the following week in public, who can also Fuck Off.)

Even if we had known our child was autistic, we did not know that for children on the spectrum, there is often a disconnect between the brain and the muscles in the bladder. Both would have been helpful knowledge. Plus, my kid was super anxious and that certainly didn't help matters.

Another day, another unfortunate situation involving my child's bladder. The location was the Cook Islands. We had decided to attend a friend's nuptials. Why? I have no idea. They weren't close friends, and hadn't I learned by now that flying with my children invariably ends with one of them inconveniently and inappropriately excreting some type of bodily fluid? How soon I forget.

So, there we were on one of those old-school public buses taking a tour around an idyllic Cook Island (to be clear, the bus was less idyllic). Which island? Don't know. Irrelevant to the story. What is relevant is the fact that Cerulean was still no closer to being able to use public washrooms and had decided in their infinite wisdom to "hold on." Midafternoon sun streamed through the dirty windows. I recall the curious sight of burial plots in the front garden of many of the modest homes on this island. What an unusual custom. Thank God my disagreeable grandmother wasn't buried in my backyard. Or front yard. Good grief. She was far enough away, be it up or down in the next world.

Staring out, I was looking at random front-yard cemeteries, and Cerulean was sitting on my lap, when I felt a warmth. In a matter of seconds their dress, my skirt, and the warm vinyl bus seat was flooded. Warm urine streamed down our legs. Of course, my kid had been holding on since breakfast (and to be fair, I don't like using public washrooms either, but at that moment, only one of us lost control of our bladder). But here's where it gets interesting. It seemed the bus had a slightly angled floor, with a gradient that veered toward the entrance and the driver. And fun fact! The quantity of wee that my child had been holding onto was enough to flow slowly but surely down under the seats in front, passing people's shoes, determined to escape, coming to rest on the stairwell at the entrance of the bus.

Another day, another apology for my child's bladder. I got up, exiting first while murmuring apologies as sweetly as I could muster. I passed two pretty, young backpackers.

Blonde, likely Norwegian. They were as horrified as they were beautiful.

"And this is why you don't have kids!" I sternly asserted as I passed them in all their youthful glory. They nodded, mute, taking in my urine-soaked floral skirt and the unfortunate ammonia scent that followed me like a bad rash. To this day I wonder if this incident affected their decision to ever have children. At the very least I'd like to think they took contraception with their boyfriends a little more seriously for a while.

I spent the remainder of the day at the resort laundry trying to clean our clothing. And just for fun, some pervert stole my underwear while it was in the dryer. I kid you not. Some weirdo in the Cook Islands was likely wearing my underwear. Why? No idea. After all, those were the days of practical underwear. How that could ever arouse the local sex pest, I just don't know.

Seven-hour road trips to my mother's became quite the ordeal. I'd have one of those plastic potties for the children that we used for toilet training. Emily, who in two days amazingly trained herself, would without a fuss happily relieve herself roadside. Poor Cerulean was so anxious that they never could manage to wee into a plastic receptacle of any type. I tried public washrooms to no avail. Now, to be fair, in outback Australia, they were often a little unpleasant. I recall one such day. They walked in, took one look around, and immediately walked back out. With a maturity that defied their age, they looked up and announced, "Yeah, I'm not using that."

The loungeroom rugs went to the "tip"—more politely termed waste transfer station. And where did they transfer it back then? A bloody big hole in the ground, that's where. Actually, every rug in the house ended up at the tip. We were blessed with hardwood floors throughout, and I was blessed with a large mop. And that mop was used daily, such were the anxieties of my eldest and their bladder.

Parenting a neurodivergent child really isn't for the faint of heart, and to my knowledge, no child—neurodivergent or otherwise—was ever born with an owner's manual.

Now as for my youngest, my son had an imaginary friend, and for a few years Mini-Man and Alex were inseparable. It should be noted that Mini-Man also made the move with us to Canada. While not uncommon, and usually a healthy stage of early childhood development, I did wonder, *Why did Mini-Man come to be?* A security blanket? A companion? Imaginary friends are known to give children a sense of control. Whatever the reason, he was certainly a regular part of the action. Perhaps Alexander felt a lack of control when exposed to his eldest sibling's meltdowns. Lord knows I did at times.

When the two elder children began school, there was an adjustment period, as there is for every younger sibling. I'll never forget the tone of perplexed disbelief when my boy, having searched the bedrooms, strode into the kitchen, looked up at me, and asked, "Where are my girls?!" with all the confidence of a Vegas pimp and the swagger and charm of an old-world movie star. With his blond hair; deep, rich, dark eyes; and perfectly symmetrical bone structure, he was constantly on the receiving end of compliments. And he missed his siblings.

Now aside from being a substitute play friend, Mini-Man was found to have other uses. Walking into the kitchen one day, I was greeted with flour and Dutch cocoa powder strewn across the floor, such that it looked like the bags had simply exploded. They were everywhere.

Alex looked me straight in the eye and asserted, "It was Mini-Man." Said with impressive confidence, I almost believed the tale, such was his convincing tone. And just to make certain that there was no confusion, with all the seriousness of a supreme court judge, Alexander earnestly stressed, "And Mummy . . . I am *not* Mini-Man."

The house was still, and I was enjoying a quiet evening over a phone call with an old friend. (Yes, this was pre-FaceTime.)

"You know, I've actually lost weight since you moved!" exclaimed Anna.

"Seriously?!" I couldn't hide my surprise. "Well, that's great!"

She laughed. "It was all your good food! But I still miss your cooking!"

Funny that my old friend missed my baking, but her waistline didn't. The children were mercifully asleep, and I was catching up with a very dear friend. We were now separated by about 5000 km and bonded through shared life experiences and our mutual weight challenges. The revelation that Anna—one of my best friends at the time—naturally began to shed weight when not eating my baked goods probably should have been something of a red flag. Perhaps at this point I could have taken a long hard look at the imbalance in my own life. After all, the cheesecake ice cream, chocolate-caramel slice, biscuits, muffins . . . all homemade, and all so very energy dense. Perhaps if I'd been breastfeeding eight babies like the infamous octomom, I may have needed this kind of caloric intake, but alas, I was breastfeeding one baby. I was not the village wetnurse, even if I was eating like I had assumed that role.

For the sake of clarity, I feel it important to mention here that there are many small but not insignificant differences between the country of my birth and my new home. You see, in Australia, a biscuit is a sweet, often crunchy, baked treat, all sugary and buttery. In North America, a biscuit is something savory, often eaten with the main meal of the day. As it turns out, both remain detrimental to my waistline.

What the women at my first-time parenting group didn't know was that I'd often bake double recipes, so that when I inevitably ate half of the cookies and cheesecake slices before playgroup, I'd have enough to take and share. At that point in my life, I exercised little self-control. My emotional eating was most certainly out of hand, and recklessly so. A vicious cycle, where the more I ate, the worse I felt. I was also not exercising regularly. The whole thing was something of a sugar-induced shitshow. And it had to change.

noodle salad

One can have no smaller or greater mastery than mastery of oneself.
—Leonardo da Vinci

I was thirty-two years old when I fainted on a plane. A long-haul flight to be exact. I'm not quite sure what possessed me to think that a holiday with a five-year-old, a three-year-old, and a one-year-old to the West Coast of North America was a good idea. Nevertheless I did, and off we went! Suffice to say, after four weeks of eating American food with its enormous portions, my jeans were more than a little tight (and they weren't small to begin with). We also traveled with Anna, her husband, her two sons, her mother, my mother, and my sister. Quite the entourage, and seriously, matching tracksuits for all would have made us easily identifiable in a crowd (perhaps not surprisingly, no one else supported this idea). After all, trying to organize five small children in an international airport—or any airport, for that matter—is like herding cats. Challenging to say the least.

Wanting to take the children to Disneyland was the initial motivation; however, I failed to realize that taking them when a little older would have made the journey a little easier. And the kids would have had a better memory of that experience.

The scene was the long-haul flight home, a brutal undertaking at the best of times. I was alternating between placing my one-year-old in the crib at the front of the plane and having him on my lap. As a parent with an infant in economy, we scored the rock star seating at the front of this section, where I could mercifully stretch my legs. So, there we were, experiencing significant turbulence on this particular fifteen-hour flight. Again, what was I thinking? I still don't know. Anyway, it turns out that when you combine sleep deprivation with dehydration, turbulence, and tight pants, fainting—it can happen. And I should know, because it happened to me. I recall feeling incredibly ill, getting up to use the bathroom, and according to the flight attendants, this is when they heard a large thud. I came to with several of them and a couple of doctors on board surrounding my dizzy form. My mother was later to recall that she heard someone exclaim, "Someone's down!"

"Was I pregnant?" they asked.

NO!

Feeling too ill to be mortified at this question, I lay there until the dizziness subsided to the point that I could stand unaided. The flight attendants later told me that they were relieved to find me both alive and young. Evidently more than one elderly passenger had collapsed on this Pacific crossing never to wake. You would think that perhaps this would have been my rock bottom. You know, the point that every food addict has when they realize that something needs to change. And change it did. But not quite yet.

It's not that I wasn't trying to lose the baby weight. I tried everything. Weight Watchers, protein drinks, walking, biking, juicing. If it had an "-ing," I'd be up for it.

I recall one very unfortunate weekend. My in-laws were visiting (again, bad timing). In my infinite wisdom, I had decided that a juice fast was the answer to my waistline, my stress, and possibly the state of the planet. After all, these diets really do promise the world, don't they? Smooth thighs, world peace, and all your problems gone!

Well, as you can probably imagine, this was not the end result. Off I marched to buy a juicer with more parts than I would ever want to wash by hand. Of course, I immediately decided the following day to begin cold turkey with my juice cleanse. No gradual easing into the regime for me! I didn't have time for that—nor did my thighs! Well, it turns out that spinach and celery juice tastes quite pleasant for the first little while (throw in some apples for sweetness—let's be clear). Unfortunately, my digestion was less than thrilled with the abrupt change to my constitution. I very quickly had an apricot and diet pills situation on my hands.

The juicer was soon after packed away and sold years later in a garage sale. I'm still hoping the new owners have more success in their juicing endeavors than I managed, and good luck to them.

I do want to stress that Weight Watchers worked. For a while. Advocating sensible eating, portion control, and healthy choices, of course it works. . . . If we can all keep it up, maintaining the changes. And that's a huge IF. Capital *I*, capital *F*. I was yet to do the emotional inner work required for real change. Permanent, transformative change. This was my downfall, and the downfall of many dieting regimes, certainly in days gone by. I'm encouraged when I see that the conversation is changing, with a greater awareness now of the psychological factors that are frequently at the root of a person's emotional eating disorder. They were certainly at the root of mine.

One final fat story from these days provided the impetus to make permanent and lasting change to my body. We were a family of skiers, and even in my most unhealthy days, I would enjoy this sport—albeit in much bigger ski pants. The scene was the bunny hill. I was teaching my four-year-old son the basics, in conjunction with his group lessons. I had learned in my youth, after all, and was a decent skier. It was only after the three back-to-back pregnancies and substantial weight gain that skiing became a whole lot of work.

I'll spare you the details of that day. Thankfully Alex was unscathed, but I injured both knees, one badly (barely able to walk on my right knee initially). Seeing a doctor the next day, I received the worst possible care that I have ever experienced in my life from a medical professional. The doctor in question was a tiny woman who took one look at my large form and made a judgment. There is no question in my mind that I was the victim of prejudice.

"Oh, just rest it a few days and you'll be fine. Some weight loss would help . . ." At that point, I received a loaded look.

And here's the thing: She didn't so much as examine my right knee, didn't touch it, didn't ask me to lift my unflattering sweatpants to assess the injury. *Nothing.* And I knew in that moment that I was being judged. Judged for being overweight. Not good enough. For being fat.

Her look said it all: *You wouldn't have hurt yourself if you weren't so overweight.* After being in the consultation room less than five minutes, I was dismissed. "Well, I'd better be getting to my next patient," she brusquely declared.

It was only a decade later, after scans ordered by my compassionate new GP, that my torn meniscus was found, with accompanying fluid on the knee. I had *torn my meniscus* that day on the ski hill! The fact that I was dismissed by the petite doctor at the walk-in clinic is both disgraceful and negligent. I failed to receive the medical attention that I required and was entitled to, as a member of the human race.

I am not alone. Countless people still are on the receiving end of discrimination by medical professionals as a result of their body size. It's disgusting, unacceptable, and it must be changed. Overweight people need compassion, and they bloody well deserve it. When did judgment and criticism ever result in positive change?

I recall one doctor, years back, warning me, "Jane, butter can power diesel engines," stressing the energy-dense nature of my favorite accompaniment to sourdough! Now I'm sure it can, but that information alone wasn't enough to prompt lasting lifestyle change. Nor was the doctor who recklessly dismissed my torn meniscus and told me to go home and rest my knee for a few days.

Enough was enough. Looking back, there are several moments in time, forever burned into my brain, that come to mind when I think about the day that I vowed to myself that I would lose the weight, and for good. The overt criticism, the humiliation, and the discomfort had taken its toll over the years. The shame and inadequacy that I felt was palpable. I was miserable. To the outside world, no one knew. I was the classic fat, happy friend. The one that many women secretly love to have around, to stand next to in a photo. After all, they looked even more petite in comparison.

Well, I was that friend, until I wasn't. I made a decision: This was not going to be my story. This time in my life became something of a turning point. Let's face it, when you fail to recognize yourself in a photo that your mother took because your physical form has changed so dramatically, it's probably a sign that something drastic needs to change. Or when people: (a) don't know that you're pregnant, or (b) a health professional can't tell when you've given birth. Well, red flag moments abounded. Time to find a hobby that didn't involve baking, perhaps.

Ironically, I'd always enjoyed exercise in my youth. My mother insisted that we played team sports, and I was always happier outside. I'd ride my bike around the neighborhood with the other kids, day in and out. There was precious little else to do. Well, the trampoline was also used daily. After all, television held little interest. There were two channels in 1989 in the outback. As a result, my childhood was lived outside—my skin now proof of too much time spent in the harsh Australian sun. The prevailing attitudes back then were very much, "Oh some sun will do you good!" My sunspots and the emerging wrinkles in my mid-forties tell a different story.

"I'm going to buy a bike trailer for my bike!" I announced to Brian soon after my momentous decision to get healthy. After all, I love riding. "And I'm joining Weight Watchers!"

To his credit, Brian was always supportive of my efforts, although he maintains that the juicer was a complete waste of money.

Agreed.

Anyway, time to move my pregnant-not-pregnant-looking form. Blessed with sunshine most days, I'd secure my little ones and head out to ride. Having begun kindergarten at this stage, my eldest was occupied during the week, allowing me to take the younger two out in our newest mode of transport. I dusted off my old bike, and off we went. It was the first of many steps on my weight loss journey that was to span many years. Nothing if not determined, slowly I began to make healthy, sustainable changes. Common sense changes. And very gradually, the weight began to fall away.

Reading Geneen Roth was another turning point. Discovering Roth around 2011 was nothing short of life changing, and I do not write these words lightly. This was also soon after the too-tight-pants, fainting-on-the-plane incident, so timing was rather helpful. I was in no rush to repeat that experience. Roth's books were instrumental in helping me—for the first time—to take a step back and begin to examine the root causes of my emotional eating. I'd simply never questioned it before. I just liked food, and I loved to cook and bake. Everyone figured I merely had a big appetite. And I did have a big appetite, but it wasn't food that I hungered for, as I would later discover. It was so much more, and the root causes of my disordered eating ran deep. Excavation was required.

A favorite film of mine has to be *As Good as It Gets*, and in 1997, the following line resonated deeply: "Some of us have great stories, pretty stories that take place at lakes with boats and friends and noodle salad. Just no one in this car. But for a lot of people, that's their story. Good times, noodle salad!" The inimitable Jack Nicholson's Melvin Udall could have been talking to me, in that scene in the blue convertible with Helen Hunt and Greg Kinnear. How I longed for summers by a lake and noodle salad and two parents who could stop shouting for five minutes. Never mind that I lived in a semi-arid desert and lakes were in short supply. As was the peace and emotional safety that every child craves in their family of origin. My disordered eating was born of an unhappy home, and it would take years to reconcile this reality.

vancouver

*Travel and change of place impart new vigour to
the mind.*

—Seneca

Marriage to a mining engineer meant a transient existence, and we were on the move again. Something of an expert now, I was beyond excited for our impending international work move. I think I began to naturally lose weight at this time, due to the inherent busyness of relocation. After all, this wasn't like other interstate moves; we were off to Canada, and I could barely hide my excitement! Hungry for adventure, I was in my element.

As far as moving goes, company moves are really very easy. Someone comes in, magically packs up your possessions, and in less than twenty-four hours, your entire life is loaded into a shipping container. I was also desperate for some breathing room. Despite its expanse, I was beginning to feel stifled in Australia. I suspect I've always had a restless soul, hungry for adventure at my core. The world is broad and wide, and I ached to explore beyond the shores of our island continent.

Our two Aussie cats also made the international move. Now for those of you who don't know, Australia has a very strict no-pets policy on all flights. It's the cargo hold for them, and as a result, I had some questions. Phoning the airline prior to departure, I recall a conversation with a rather bemused gentleman. I was curious. Would they be given access to water? Clean litter? Food? Was the area that they were to be transported in under lighting or in the dark?

"Why? Can your cat read?!" he chortled.

After his laughter died down, I discovered that although they usually don't die (despite being locked in a plastic crate for over twenty-four hours door to door), they aren't given food or water on long haul flights out of Australia. After all, the air on these planes is recycled and circulating throughout. The no food policy minimizes the chance that my cat would take a dump and the entire plane would be forced to endure the smell. Makes sense. You can imagine my shock when I began flying within North America and two rows ahead someone is patting their cat. And who's controlling their bowels? Does the cat know not to poo mid-flight?

"What the fuck?!" was Emily's initial reaction. My children are wide-eyed to this day when there's a cat near them on a flight. Given that we are a family of elderly cat ladies at heart, it's all rather exciting. And I suppose it does distract from the inedible food, uncomfortable seating, and screaming children (mercifully not my own anymore).

"Excuse me . . ."

Brian and I both turned to see a well-dressed older gentleman sitting directly behind us in his economy row seat, mildly cramped and uncomfortable, as we were. "I just wanted to tell you that your kids have been great, you should be very proud. When my wife and I sat down, we were a little worried, being directly behind three kids, but they've been terrific!" He chuckled.

I was touched. "Oh, thank you! How lovely of you to say so! You know, our kids have flown quite a bit. They know the deal." I shrugged, offering a friendly we're-all-in-this-together smile. We were into hour fourteen of a fifteen-hour direct Sydney–Vancouver flight that day, blessedly nearly done.

Now what happened next can't possibly have been a coincidence. No sooner had I bid the friendly couple good day and turned back to assume my cramped position, my sweet little Emily took one look at me and proceeded to vomit, violently expelling the contents of her stomach with impressive force. The apple really doesn't fall far, does it?! The older couple behind us were aghast at the irony of it all.

The flight attendant didn't bother to hide her distain any more than my poor little girl could hide the contents of her stomach. Given the crap that they served up in economy and called food, quite frankly, I'm surprised that more people didn't regurgitate their meals.

I confess to having eaten the dreadful economy food myself. The cold, stale bread roll. Why? To escape, to pass the time. Old habits dying hard, and let's be fair, who wouldn't want to escape a long-haul economy flight? Barely tolerable at the best of times, this quickly descended into the flight from hell. Much like the stale roll filled with a rather limp lettuce leaf and single slice of dreadful processed cheese. Ahh . . . cattle class. "We're not happy until you're not happy!" Surely this was their unofficial motto?

I think my youngest put it best when, in the midst of deplaning (a clumsy term if ever there was one), he looked on at the business class area with a mixture of awe and exhaustion. "Mummy, next time we fly, can we *please* sit at the front of the plane? Mummy, they have *beds*!"

"Oh honey, I'm sorry, but no. No, we can't."

My four-year-old was less than impressed with my response, and who can blame him?

Now, here's a fun fact for you. When you land in a new country on a work visa, it turns out that the whole getting through security thing takes just a little longer. And bear in mind, this is just off the back of Emily's power spew from hell. We were done. Reeking mildly of stale vomit, immigration then proceeded to interrogate us as to our plans. The highlight of the day had to be the line in the mountain of official government paperwork that was stated clearly on my visa, allowing us to remain in the country. It read, "I am not authorized to engage in any paid employment, including work in the sex trade."

Got it. Given that I reeked of vomit, was mildly disheveled, not to mention standing at the immigration desk with three small children, did I look like I was about to engage in illegal sex-trade work? Seriously?! (Did he think I needed money to feed the children?) I barely had the energy to walk to the baggage carousel. I certainly didn't have the energy to satisfy the needs of the randy men of Canada. Let's face it, my husband would have been lucky if he got laid anytime soon.

"Where are they sending you?" the young customs official asked when he saw that we were there thanks to the mining industry. Expecting that we were in transit, en route to some tiny mining community up north, I imagine he was curious.

"We're staying here, in Vancouver, for a couple of years," I told him. Weary, I managed a smile.

And then, with a look I've never forgotten, he said with certainty in his smile, "Oh . . . you're not going home."

And he was right. The customs official was of course referring to Australia, and here I am, twelve years later and counting.

The adjustment was challenging. An October move from one hemisphere to the other meant back-to-back winters. One glorious week of sun upon our arrival, and then it started raining. It stopped the following May. Something of a welcome to Vancouver in that initial blissful week, the children were lured into a false sense of meteorological security. Prior to leaving, we had been warned by a colleague of Brian's. "Vancouver has two seasons. Winter and August!"

More than a decade later, this is slowly but surely changing, with climate change wreaking havoc on this temperate rainforest. Perhaps if I stay long enough, I'll have the climate of my youth right here in the Pacific Northwest. Oppressive heat and wildfires in parts of Canada now certainly remind one of home. It would all be rather comforting if it wasn't so devastating.

Practical needs were sorted that first year, most being tedious, all of them time-consuming.

"Hi there! We have an appointment to open a new bank account," said Brian to the primly dressed lady behind the desk.

"Certainly, sir. Right this way." We were then ushered into a small, forgettable room and greeted by a friendly, well-dressed man who looked to have been on the planet for around thirty years.

It was 2012. We had just emigrated to Canada, and we needed, among a million other things, a Canadian credit card. As I was to find out momentarily, this process was akin to time travel. No, our credit scores at home were not recognized here, despite both countries being members of the Commonwealth. No, we couldn't lease a car or have a small loan. No, we couldn't have a credit limit even close to the limit on our Australian cards. No, no, no. This was, I'll remind you, despite my then-husband's rather large six-figure income (thank you, mining industry). The following conversation I have never forgotten.

With our three young children beside us, the bank employee looked to Brian and asked, no word of a lie, "Now, sir, would you like your wife to have the same credit limit on her companion card as yours?"

Blank face, quite serious. I'd like to point out that this conversation took place *in front of me*.

"Ahh . . . yes?" To be fair, Brian wasn't sure what to say to this question.

"Are you *sure*?" asked Bank Man, surprise in his pene-trating gaze, silently emphasizing his question. I kid you not.

Now, I was suspicious for a moment that my husband may have been trying to discreetly pass a note under the table to Bank Man, reading NO! However, he did not.

I was in shock. Was this 2012 or 1912? Good Lord. Had the feminist movement really only taken us this far? In this moment I realized that, not only was the patriarchy alive and well, evidently in Vancouver it was thriving.

The challenges didn't end there. Driver's licenses, hous-ing, it went on. And as I was to learn some years later, my lack of credit rating would prove problematic. You see, like many housewives of that time, everything was in Brian's name. There was simply no record of me in Canada, even after many years. I barely existed. No tax returns, no credit scores. Nothing.

My eldest struggled the most that winter. In hindsight, seasonal affective disorder had likely set in. The weight of parenting our neurodivergent (still undiagnosed) child began to take a toll on the marriage. How could it not? We were both exhausted, parenting had become a daily battle with Cerulean, and we'd retreat at the end of a long day like weary soldiers returning from battle to the dugout to grab a few precious hours of sleep before awaking to do it all again the following day. Overwhelmed, food was still my refuge on a stressful day. Change was happening, but slowly.

And then Alexander began kindergarten. Suddenly, all three children were occupied, educated between the hours of 9:00 a.m. and 3:00 p.m. Feeling like I could finally breathe for the first time in a decade, I resumed walking. A daily commitment to myself. Still determined to lose the remainder of the baby weight, I'd walk. What began as a healthier escape has now become as necessary to my well-being as water and oxygen. An essential daily need.

A quick fix is never the answer to a decades-long battle with emotional eating. How can it be? I was attempting to heal from the outside. The answers began when I looked inward. Looking back, my healing journey began with walking, with Geneen Roth's books, and with the introduction of yoga. What I didn't know at the time is that yoga is an extremely powerful pathway into the body. I was reconnecting my mind with my body after a disconnect of more than two decades. I was coming home. Of course, I didn't realize this at that point. I just realized that after a family yoga session, the entire family was calm, grounded, happier—and mercifully quieter!

I was on the very precipice of reclaiming my body as I finally began to nurture and connect with myself somatically. My journey home had begun. Mostly flat walking initially, I then incorporated hills. The dopamine started flowing. I didn't know that either then. I just knew that I felt better after a walk and was far more able to tackle the challenges that come with parenting three young children in a foreign country, while the entirety of our extended family was on the other side of the Pacific Ocean.

Sadly, the stress continued to take a toll on the marriage. There were other factors of course, and too intimate to be shared here, they will therefore forever remain private. In those early years in Canada, our marriage began to show the strain, so slowly at first that neither of us were aware of what would come next.

Initially unaware that my marriage was imploding, I couldn't sleep. I stopped eating. Once a good sleeper, I was suddenly awake at 2:00 a.m., finding Brian, as always, working on the laptop. We kept odd hours. He would sleep after dinner, wake at midnight, and get back to work. I'd cook, clean, and retire to bed night after night to lie there awake. Sleep eluded me.

Brian was endlessly patient. He was also concerned. Something was amiss, and he didn't know how to fix it. In that typically male and very sincere way, he wanted to fix things. It's what men do. But I couldn't be fixed, and I knew it.

change

Parting is all we know of heaven, and all we need of hell.

—Emily Dickenson

I was thirty-eight when I left my husband. It was the single hardest thing that I have ever done.

Jan, my ever-pragmatic mother, shared the following wisdom: "Most women leave a marriage because their husband is abusive, or a cheater. Brian is neither of those things!" She was perplexed, but I ask: Is the bar really this low? Should a woman remain unhappily married because she isn't beaten?!

We were children when we met, and with youthful enthusiasm I threw myself into our relationship, engagement, and marriage with a naiveté typical of my age. To this day Brian doesn't agree that we were too young to make such a momentous commitment. But ultimately, I was still figuring out who I was. We both were. Isn't this what our twenties should be for? Growth, exploration, adventure, maturing? At twenty I was certainly still a child in the world—and a child with daddy issues at that. Of course, I married the first responsible man who looked sideways at me! He was reliable, sensible, and on track to have a solid career. He was everything my father wasn't. I was certainly infatuated with my handsome

71

boyfriend. I probably even thought that I was in love. It wasn't until 2015 that I knew with certainty that while I loved my husband and the father of my three children, I needed more.

"You've always been more than enough for me, Jane."

Brian didn't understand. Perhaps this highlighted our differences more than anything else. We didn't understand each other. The lack of connection didn't bother him; what we had was enough. I disagreed. I knew at the core of my being that I would forever yearn for more.

"Jane, slow down!" Brian was banging on the passenger seat dashboard, sounding far too much like his father. I was driving, in control (where I've always preferred to be). Brian has long told me that I drive like a man, and I've long maintained that he drives like an old lady. Now this caution does have its benefits, as he now drives our children around solo with only the gods to protect them all. But when married, arguments over our driving styles abounded. In hindsight, this was an excellent metaphor for our marriage, and perhaps gives a little insight into the way we lived.

My father briefly taught me to drive—another rare attempt at parenting. He, too, concluded that I didn't drive like a girl, and frankly I was too young and naive to take offense to the comment at the time.

Willingly, Brian and I shouldered massive responsibility at a very young age. Mortgage at twenty-five, babies—responsibilities that we thought we were ready for. I desperately wanted a traditional, happy home for our young children. Yearning for the stability that my own childhood lacked, we both threw ourselves into our roles for the next decade or so. You see, we were still growing up, alongside our young family—one of the many challenges of starting a family at twenty-five. And it worked for a time, until it didn't.

Things began to crumble. Music became my new escape, slowly beginning to replace the comfort food that I had relied upon for decades—up until now. I was in the middle of another day of laundry, lost in another world, when Brian walked downstairs. In no possible earthly coincidence, the lyrics to Imagine Dragons's "Demons" hit me, haunting through my headphones, singing my life. And I cried. Again.

On my hardwood rocking chair sat Ted, the shaggy, stuffed teddy bear. This beautiful piece of furniture, beloved and frequented when nursing, was now the home of once-worn clothes in our bedroom. Ted was witness to our crumbing marriage. Stoic and confused, he lay upside down on my rocking chair, perfectly reflecting the discombobulated world that we now inhabited.

I moved out in the spring of 2016. Brian refused to move out, and fair enough, I suppose. After all, he didn't want out.

"If you want out of this marriage, Jane, then you can be the one to move out. You live in a basement suite."

And so I did. I remember the moment all too well. Lying in the rented basement suite on the uncomfortable mattress that had once been our guest bed, my mind was spinning and showed no sign of slowing. I was alone, had no money, and had left my husband weeks before. As I reflected on the affluent family and owners living upstairs, I couldn't help but think, *What the hell happened to my life?* I no longer recognized it. Five years prior I was the mother of the family in the beautiful home in Australia. It was I who would extend charity to others. Money was something that just came in, and there was always more than enough.

On that day in the basement, I had opened a bank account in my own name for the first time in Canada and deposited a toonie ($2 for people who aren't familiar with the reference). I had zero credit rating. There was simply no record of me. After all, everything had been in my husband's name. The car, the insurance. I was somebody's wife. I was somebody's mother, daughter, sister. But who was I? Marriage had defined my adult life up until this moment. The patriarchy was alive and thriving, and I was living proof.

Auntie Sue disapproved. Wholeheartedly. "Marriage is for life. You work through your problems. Divorce is unacceptable!"

This logic is flawed. While I agree that attempting to work through one's marital problems is typically a good thing, should we also be tethered permanently to this person for life due to a promise made too young? The judgment hurt. My new Canadian friend, Sensible Susan, was right. Marriage is a daily choice.

In the beginning, it was one day at a time. Then one week. Then one month. I got a part-time job. I decided to go back to school—both needing and wanting a career at this point. In those early days I couldn't eat (great for my perpetual diet but not much else). I wasn't sleeping. There were too many unanswered questions. The children were thrust into the madness of a two-two-five-five schedule that some of you know all too well. For anyone familiar with the darkness of separation, you will recognize the hell I describe here on these pages. And the children were my primary concern. Always.

Crying every day, I tried in vain to shield my children from the grief. They were also witness to their father's grief. Deeper, I know, as this decision was thrust upon him, entirely out of his control. For a man, for any man, the loss of control must have been frightening. After all, ours was a traditional, 1950s-style union from the beginning. Suddenly the balance of power had shifted, as if the northern hemisphere was now the southern, our world forever and permanently changed beyond recognition. My autonomous decision left me with newfound control, and my estranged husband found himself, for the first time, without. His world was upside down. Everybody's was.

The basement suite was dark, as basements are apt to be. The Bunker, I called it. After all, bunkers are traditionally a place of safety, a refuge, and of course underground, where I most definitely was. There was a feeling of groundlessness in those early days, despite being surrounded by earth quite literally. I craved the sunlight, like only an Australian can. Vancouver rain depressing in its frequency, that spring was unusually wet, even by Vancouver standards. And somber, reflecting the mood of the time. If you've experienced a separation after many years, you'll know the feeling well. Horrific and surreal in equal measure. Being the one to make this monumental decision didn't make it any easier. My estranged husband became depressed, angry.

I became fearful for Brian's well-being. His thoughts became quite dark in those early days. Extended family and friends were shocked; no one saw this coming. In hindsight, neither did Brian. Against all advice of my closest confidantes, I refused to retain a lawyer. Brian was deeply wounded and implored me to reconsider, hoping for reconciliation. Should I return for the children? Another decade until they're grown? Despite wavering, I knew the answer. Staying wasn't fair to either of us. I didn't know it yet, but my course was set in a different direction. Hungry for life, for independence, for experiences and adventure that I couldn't have yet imagined.

The Bunker was challenging. And foreign. Basement suites are practically nonexistent in Australia. We have no need for them. In Vancouver they are an essential piece of the housing landscape in what is the second-most expensive city in Canada to reside in, and one of the most unaffordable globally, when taking into account average incomes. Typically inhabited by students and newly separated men, my kids and I joined their ranks out of necessity.

My children were disoriented, no one more than my eldest. Cerulean had been diagnosed with obsessive compulsive disorder at this point and was medicated. Another agonizing decision. . . . We'd tried therapy alone first to no avail. The combination of medication and therapy, on the other hand, worked. Years later we were told that this was all classic spectrum behavior, the autism specialist hinting at a former misdiagnosis. Nevertheless, this is what they were diagnosed with at the time.

Children at school were vicious, the mean girls pulling their long blonde hair and poking them, ruthless in their cruelty. Cerulean would return from school, collapse on the rug in the basement, and sob. Heartbreaking to witness as a parent. And then one day they snapped.

Mother was visiting at the time (thankfully, in hindsight). I can't recall the argument, but I do recall Cerulean's screaming, my child throwing water in my face, all over myself, the floor, and several pieces of technology. Their siblings were crying, and I am not proud of what happened next. Like my father before me I grabbed them and gave their bottom a fair whack with my open hand. I felt sick. Remorse flooded my body, but it was too late. They screamed.

"Mummy, that's child abuse! I'm phoning the police!" And of course, being my child, that's exactly what they did.

"Jane, they've called the police," my mother said, horrified and less calm than I at this point.

Now, I have a blessedly calm disposition under stress. (I'm still not sure who I inherited this useful trait from, but I'm grateful.) I look at Mum and respond, matter-of-factly, "Well, I'll just explain the situation. I have a medicated child, and I'm in the middle of a separation. My child isn't abused, locked in some cupboard under the stairs, for God's sake."

Now Cerulean had just been given their first iPhone about this time, a common move made by newly separated parents. Suddenly our kids needed a direct line to the other parent, and who had a landline anymore? We certainly didn't. In any event, you can probably see where this is going. I spent the remainder of the evening, calmly on the phone and in person with the police officer, fortunately able to convince them that my child was not a victim of child abuse. The entire experience was agonizing. To their credit, the lovely female police officer spent the rest of the evening with Cerulean, explaining what 911 is meant for, and what constitutes an emergency and abuse. Thankfully my child was dressed in clean clothing at the time, and it was evident that they were loved, fed, clothed, and generally cared for in a clean (if currently underground) home. This day went down in history as quite the shitshow.

"What matters most is how well you walk through the fire."

Charles Bukowski wasn't kidding. I didn't have a choice. You give up that freedom when you become a parent. I was going through hell and had to keep going. We all were at that point.

Life eventually settled down a little, the children adjusting to the new normal, my eldest stabilized on their medication.

I also ached, with a deep sadness and longing. I was lonely and ached to have that connection that I witnessed amongst some couples. You know the type. Across a room they'd share a glance, a knowing smile. And they'd just know what the other thought, felt, desired. There was nothing but a deep sadness that remained when I realized that I had never shared that with my husband of thirteen years. We lacked that small but significant connection, the shared glances. And I ached for that depth of understanding and connection with another human. And I cried. Deep, wracking sobs as I sat on my Craigslist couch in the basement of someone else's home. I cried for the good, kind man whom I was hurting. For the children, whose lives would never be the same. And I cried for myself, because I knew that Brian and I had come as far as we could together on our journey. I knew that our marriage was over. I had begun a transformation.

"You've changed," said Brian. Well, yes, I suppose I had. I was certainly a great deal smaller at this point. But it was so much more than that. I had a newfound confidence. I no longer suffered with anxiety. A stressful day didn't result in twelve hours of bedrest and the violent emptying of my stomach. I had changed. Don't we all change as we mature and evolve?

I didn't know where this yearning would take me or why, but I somehow just knew that a new chapter lay ahead. The thing is, leaving Brian would have been so much easier if he wasn't such a good man. Those days were horrific, and mercifully they have passed, the pain softened with the inevitable passage of time.

trouble

Love is a serious mental disease.

—Plato

I first saw him at my children's school fair. He was laughing (ironically with his ex-wife). She was very pretty in a yes-and-I-know-it sort of way. His head thrown back, confident, charismatic. Charming? I had no doubt, as he would later confirm. Isn't it interesting, the way that some people have the ability to draw a person toward them with their magnetism, an almost tangible gravity? This powerful ability dangerous in the wrong hands. And even more dangerous when the woman drawn into their orbit is equal parts innocence, playfulness, and recklessness.

Sebastian became a dangerous obsession, slowly at first. Our children shared a classroom one year, and a brief friendship; we shared a very clear interest in learning about each other, coupled with an undeniable chemistry. Playdates became an opportunity to chat.

Having traveled far along my weight loss journey at this stage, I was discovering for the first time, at the age of thirty-eight, just exactly how much power a woman could wield over a man with just the right pair of jeans. It was intoxicating, this new ability of mine. I'd suddenly gone from the frumpy mother at school pickup to the pretty parent with the charming accent and the tight derriere. I worked bloody hard to reclaim my health and fitness. The deeper rewards weren't external however, despite the pleasure that I felt in wearing a new pair of jeans that were, for the first time, truly comfortable. The increased energy and ease that I found in my new body far outweighed any appreciation of my external silhouette.

Anyway, as it happened, Sebastian also had an appreciation for my newly toned figure. Texts were innocent at first. Organizing kids and so forth. Then playful. Then a line was crossed. I still recall the pounding of my heartbeat. The mild flirtation continued. We found opportunities for our paths to conveniently cross through our children's friendship. For the first time in too many years, I began to care about the state of my hair. Dusting off the hairdryer (after finding it), the days of the week became the days that he would be at school pickup, and the days he wouldn't. I quickly became obsessed. And for the first time in my life, I felt alive to the very core of my being. Desired, I awoke. Drunk on infatuation . . . it was intoxicating.

Every woman knows this moment. For some it happens very young, in that dreamy innocence of youth. For myself it was much later, a world away from the dusty hometown of my childhood. Perhaps appropriate that I had to travel so very far to find myself. And at the age of thirty-eight, I fell in love. Initially infatuation, this rapidly intensified—equal parts reckless, obsessive, dangerous. And let's face it, I'd never been one for moderation (that lesson would come later). For the very first time, I couldn't eat. I couldn't sleep. And for an emotional eater with a very disordered eating problem, this was no small thing. Never before had I lost my appetite, save one summer in my childhood with an unfortunate illness—and of course the initial separation from Brian. Was it measles that summer? Perhaps. I recall laying under my grandmother's air conditioner in the hallway and overhearing her brusque comments. My mother had offered me ice cream, and I had declined.

"Well, she really must be sick if she doesn't want ice cream!"

To be fair, it was probably the first time I had ever said no to ice cream.

The second was Sebastian.

"Never sleep with someone whose troubles are worse than your own."

Indeed, Nelson Algren. The late American writer and winner of the National Book Award in 1949 was correct, and it's safe to say that I've broken this rule more than once. Algren's sage advice would have been useful post-separation, though no doubt I would have ignored it anyway. Never one to allow common sense to trump passion when it comes to matters of the heart, I dove headlong into my not-quite-fatal attraction. And it was delicious. Of course, he broke my naive, reckless heart, like only the charming Sebastian could. Completely, thoroughly, and without care. Himself, thoughtless in his pursuit and subsequent disposal of me; myself, newly separated and wild with my heart. Perhaps I deserved this karma? After all, I'd sworn in a church to remain by Brian's side until death, and I broke that promise. Was the universe punishing me? A reminder that I had broken this promise? Perhaps. And when had my life become a Taylor Swift song? 2016, apparently.

"Jane, most of us learn these lessons in our twenties. While we were all out partying, you were pregnant and breastfeeding! You're just learning these lessons a little later." Kellie, my measured Libra best friend, right as always.

"I know, and you're right. Thanks, Kells."

Sobbing, I was a hot mess. My face wet with a million tears, FaceTime bearing witness to life lessons that I was learning two decades too late. My best friend turned therapist half a world away, and invariably patient with me. I just wouldn't have survived those early years of freedom without my oldest friend. How she tolerated my frequent emotional communications back then is still beyond me, and I am forever grateful and indebted to her. The woman deserves a medal.

"Mummy, are they happy tears or sad tears?" Emily asked.

My precious second child, my baby girl. And my heart broke at this question. Again. So many sad tears in those early days. My child learned early on to be on the lookout for grief.

Emmy has the innate ability to read the room like a barometer reads the air pressure—my emotional weathervane. It developed over time due to living with an autistic, and often volatile, elder sibling. Emmy had to be on alert. Constantly on the lookout for any discord, she knew that her emotional and sometimes physical safety relied upon this. Prior to Cerulean beginning medication, they were at times physically aggressive, and no member in the family was spared this hostility. Had I any spare cash, stocks in Kleenex would have been a wise investment—such was the quantity of tissues that were required that first year.

Divorce impacts children. Anyone who says otherwise is an idiot. Then again, an unhappy home also impacts children. Looking back, our home wasn't an unhappy one; however, I had reached a point where I was no longer happy to be married. I no longer wanted the union that I had chosen, despite Brian being a decent bloke. I also had to ask myself some very hard questions. Would I want my children to remain unhappy, due to vows that they had promised another? Well, no, of course not.

Sensible Susan is right. My ever-practical friend (also the child of a divorce) shared the following: "I wake up every day and choose to be married, Jane. For me, marriage is a daily choice." She also pointed out that divorce is financial suicide. Sensible advice indeed. Never one to choose practicality over my heart, I knew that I would never remain in any situation for financial gain.

"Money comes and money goes. You can always make more of it, Jane." Mar's wisdom—a former paramour and now dear friend. And he's right. There's certainly no shortage of it on the planet, and despite being wildly uneven in its distribution, I reasoned that money was out there. Ever the optimist, I'd just figure out a way to have some of it make its way into my humble bank account.

education

To affect the quality of the day,
that is the highest of arts.

—Henry David Thoreau

"I 'm going back to school!" I announced with enthusiasm to my Vancouver confidantes, also known as the First Wives Club.

I knew that I both wanted and needed a career, that much was clear in my own mind. I wanted to contribute positively in some way in society, to the best of my abilities. I'd already added an extra three humans to our crowded planet, so I decided that perhaps it was time to be of service to a few of them. Becoming a counselor would fulfil that requirement while allowing myself the flexibility and freedom that I needed with my schedule as I balanced work and motherhood as a solo parent. I dislike the term single mother (despite being exactly that), as it conjures negative connotations; pity and disdain come to mind, and that's a hard pass.

"I think it's a terrible idea, Jane. You'll just tell women to leave their husbands!"

Wow. Thanks, Brian. My estranged husband made his feelings quite clear on the subject of my future career. What he didn't know was that I would later develop an interest in working with disordered eating clients through my practice. Not exactly surprising.

Prior to the separation, Brian and I had tried marriage counseling. The first therapist he didn't like, the second I didn't like, and the third was excellent. Despite not saving our marriage, I did come to the realization that I wanted to pursue a career in counseling. I discovered that there were a lot of bad counselors out there, and that there seemed to be a gap in the market for good ones. I just knew in my bones that this was the next step for me.

Tuition was prohibitive, and as I wasn't yet a citizen of this fine country, student loans were not an option. We hadn't yet sold our enormous family home in Australia at this point, so I had no access to any real money. I had to learn to budget, and fast.

From the very beginning of the separation, I had something of a cash flow problem. Ever resourceful and optimistic, I decided to do something about it. Having agreed to a humble private child support arrangement that lasted many years, I was acutely aware of my need for funds.

Why did I agree?

Guilt.

So much guilt over leaving. After all, Brian had fought hard to try and save the marriage, and I hadn't forgotten this. I therefore refused the legal route. Brian was angry and depressed. I knew that advocating for myself financially might tip him over the edge of a cliff to which he was dangerously close. After all, it was never about the money. I wanted my freedom, and I had it. It was therefore time for a plan.

Taking a casual position in a toy store was both humbling and empowering. I made $11 an hour—yes, I wish that was a typo. My estranged husband pulled in large six figures, and despite this discrepancy, the feeling of receiving my first paycheck in over a decade was one of pride. Being treated poorly by entitled patrons of the store? Not so much.

I started to make decisions. School was the obvious choice. Having completed two undergrad degrees in Australia prior to my marriage, I knew that this was the perfect springboard into postgraduate studies in Canada. I needed to make real money, and a career seemed the natural choice. I didn't think I was cut out for a life of crime, and despite my somewhat husky voice, I had no interest in becoming a phone sex worker, so further education did seem prudent. It was time to rebuild my life from the ground up. Well, from the basement up really, given my current location.

The children and I eventually moved from the basement into a run-down (but pleasant enough) old rental house with more bedrooms. It was walking distance to their elementary school and the local village shops. This was essential, as I was yet to own my own car. Legally separated at this point, Brian insisted that we share the one family car to save money. The car would follow the children. Having precious little money of my own and still worried for his mental state, I reluctantly agreed. It was madness, yet I worried for my children when they weren't under my roof. What mother doesn't? I figured, *Keep the peace with Brian while he also begins to rebuild his life, and the kids will be happier for it.* And so, I walked, often with an umbrella, Vancouver being the temperate rainforest that it is. And on the bright side, the walking certainly helped as I continued to shed those last few pounds.

During those years I went back to school, completed my MA, worked part-time to bring in a little cash, and hosted international students to help pay the bills (tax-free income in British Columbia, and possibly the only thing they don't tax in this overtaxed province). I was suddenly living with five children, three of them looking a lot like me. These were happy, chaotic days. My children were exposed to different cultures and languages. We had our own United Nations of Australians, Germans, Italians, and an Austrian, Columbian, and Brazilian in the mix, plus my Canadian girlfriends and whomever I happened to be dating at the time. The dinner table became an interesting time, no more so than when, in the year after the Germans beat the Brazilians in the World Cup, we hosted boys from both countries. It was a happy time, save the day of their rematch!

There was the weekly Costco run, and the cooking. So much cooking. I spent an inordinate amount of time in that little rental kitchen, barefoot and decidedly not pregnant. Thank the Lord. I had more than my hands full with other people's children. My mother's greatest fear was that I would fall pregnant to some Tinder Swindler (this was the time of online dating). Not bloody likely. They took one look at my life and ran. One man asked, "You have how many children at home?!" A career man himself, divorced with no children, he quickly friend-zoned me the day following our shared drinks. The thought of dating a woman with five children in her care clearly sent him into some kind of panic.

Thank you. Next.

Standing in the airport arrivals hall, I surveyed the scene. The emotionality was infectious. Raw happiness never fails to move me, and I wonder, why can't we always express love so easily?

I looked up to see that the Qantas flight I awaited was early to land. Will wonders never cease! Anna was visiting, having made the massive trek from Perth, Australia. No small feat given the distance from the West Coast of Australia to my new Canadian West Coast abode. I was elated—and appreciative of the effort. I missed my dear friend; I still do. The thing is, very quickly after landing, Anna realized that my new life was one of organized chaos. Organized, to be sure, but consistently hectic.

On the day before her departure, one of my children had returned home from school with a very sprained ankle. Another student was on crutches at the time. Another two were deep in a heated debate. I had a paper to write, dinner to cook (for six including Anna, who for a grown-up, is a ridiculously fussy eater), and a house to clean. And someone needed homework help. I was exhausted.

Sitting in the lounge room, my dear friend looked over at me, briefly lifting her eyes from her cell phone. The look was one of horror and amazement.

"I have no idea how you do this, Jane."

Yes, well, you and me both.

Anna, God bless my sweet only-child friend, had other concerns. You see, she'd bid on an upgrade with points, hoping to secure a business-class seat and lie-flat bed for the journey home. Hers were champagne problems if ever there were any. As she went back to staring at her phone (sitting next to her oversized Louis Vuitton travel bag, no less), I heard a holler from upstairs. I suspected the argument was over the last coveted piece of banana bread.

"Mummmmmmmyyyyyyyyy!"

Standing to investigate, I sighed, and at this very moment Anna looked up and exclaimed, overjoyed, "I got an upgrade!"

united nations

It is time for parents to teach young
people early on that in diversity there is
beauty and there is strength.

—Maya Angelou

My international students became an extension of our family, and I loved these children like my own. Of course, none of them were really children anymore. The German students were surprisingly mature, mini-adults without the legal status. My dear Antonio, on the other hand, was very much the absent-minded professor. I'd like to preface these stories by sharing that Antonio has grown into a fine young man, now very capable and pursuing postgraduate studies in Brazil. When he came to me, though, he was still in the process of maturing, and I quickly found myself in the role of mothering another teen.

My first opportunity to provide guidance came early in the semester. You see, Antonio had decided to go to a party. Given his age, the homestay company allowed a 1:00 a.m. curfew. He was, after all, an adult—almost.

The scene was the lounge room, mother had just flown in, and we were enjoying a quiet nightcap with my steady boyfriend of the moment. Life was pleasant. And then I heard a key rustle at the door.

More rustling.

"That must be Antonio!" said Jan.

"That's odd," said the boyfriend. "He seems to be having trouble with the door. I'll check."

Excellent. More bonus points. Men really do have their uses at times. After all, it's 1:00 a.m., and if there's some oddball on my porch, I'd rather not be the one to confront him at this hour.

"Ahh, Jane, I think you'd better come up here."

Hmmm.

I wander upstairs, curious. Curiosity quickly turned to bewilderment. There's my dear homestay son, swaying. Eyes glassy, vomit down not one, but both pant legs. Still swaying, he stumbles through the entrance and into the kitchen, incoherent. Evidently thirsty, my Antonio attempts to turn on the tap . . . assistance is required. The rest of the evening went much as you can imagine when you are trying to assist a drunk seventeen-year-old safely into his bathroom (he barely made it).

The following day (again after working my crappy job) I had the unfortunate task of taking Antonio to the local supermarket to rent a carpet cleaner. You see, in his drunken stupor, he'd gotten back out of bed, vomited all over the carpet, his bed, his laptop, and part of the wall. It was something to behold.

The only thing more impressive were his outraged parents, shouting at him in Portuguese over FaceTime, and I swear, no one has lived until they've heard angry Brazilian parents shouting in Portuguese. I have no idea what they said—I didn't want to know. I had a room to clean. And they had every reason to be outraged. You see, Antonio had returned home early that morning sans backpack. And unbeknownst to me, that backpack contained his wallet, credit cards, homestay information, and photocopies of his passport. In short, everything. Why did he take all of this on his vodka-drinking bender? I still don't know. What I do know is that it took months for Antonio to obtain another credit card. As for his laptop, it was dead in the water. His parents refused to replace it. Fair punishment, I guess. Kindly, Brian took pity on the young man and loaned him a work laptop. The running joke for months was that somewhere in Vancouver there was now a tourist wandering around, quite pleased with himself, sporting a new coat and backpack purchased in Sao Paulo, Brazil.

"Ahh, Jane, I think I need a doctor . . ." said Antonio as he stood before me in that little rental house kitchen. He looked about as worn as the faded laminate on the aging doors and benchtops that had also seen better days. Gingerly, slightly bent in the midsection, Antonio looked over at me (looking much like I did after consuming too many diet pills at age seventeen). He'd phoned late in the afternoon to tell me that he had a worsening stomachache.

"Oh dear. Okay! Let's get our coats on." I forced a smile, sighing inwardly. Now this may read as uncaring. I wasn't. What I was, was tired. I'd just returned from my $11-an-hour pretend job (it may have risen to $12 at this stage). It was also snowing steadily outside (an early winter snowstorm, more common now with our extreme Vancouver weather), and I needed to cook dinner for the remaining four—and Antonio, if he didn't die. So off we traipsed, out to the car through the snow, in search of an open walk-in medical clinic.

"I'm so sorry, we don't accept this travel insurance. You'll need cash up front."

I looked blankly at the lady behind the desk, unimpressed. "I see."

At this point Antonio was fast resembling the pallor of the falling snow outside. So of course, we were sent to another clinic to try our luck. Through the snow I drove, with great caution given that Vancouver all but grinds to a halt when the snow falls. Most people don't have snow tires, and people simply don't know how to drive in the snow. Fender benders abound. The tow truck companies do a roaring trade. *How excited must they be when the snow falls*, I wondered. And then I wracked my brain. *Where to next?*

"I suggest you try the hospital emergency department. They may see him. Where is he from again?"

"Brazil. On exchange. Here's his travel insurance." I pulled out a stack of papers that mercifully weren't lost during the Drunk Antonio episode.

"Well, I'm very sorry, however, we're completely full tonight and not accepting any more patients."

Could she not have mentioned this earlier?!

Jacket zipped back up, I pushed open the heavy door to a fresh blast of snow, suddenly more awake in the frigid night air.

"Let's go. It's okay, Antonio. I'll find you a doctor." I looked over, trying to reassure my very unwell Brazilian boy. The poor kid. He really did look ill. Having texted with his parents, they feared a serious illness and insisted he see a doctor. I agreed.

If the snowy driving wasn't challenge enough, finding parking at the local hospital certainly was. Where on Earth do they expect sick people to leave their vehicles? I wondered, *Was this a ploy to deter potential patients?* I was sure some of the less unwell simply give up and go home. Now given that Antonio looked increasingly ill, and he was in my care for ten months, I thought it best I get him looked at by a medical professional.

Parking secured, we traipsed through the deepening snow like weary travelers in search of an inn for the night, headed with single-minded purpose in the direction of the bright red EMERGENCY sign. We were met with another nurse, and another set of insurance questions.

"No, he's not a citizen of this country." (Did I look like his mother?)

"No, we've tried a walk-in clinic. They sent us here."

"No, we phoned another. There was a two-day wait."

"I see. Well, to see a doctor will be $1200 upfront."

Canadian? Was she serious? Sure, $1200 Brazilian reais I could find, but Canadian dollars? Negative, Houston.

"I'm sorry, what?" Antonio and I both stared blankly at the intake nurse.

"Jane, I don't have access to that cash." Well, that made two of us. I certainly didn't back then. These were the post-separation days. I barely had access to my cats (they lived with Brian). I certainly didn't have any access to marital funds (my backup plan was to phone my mother for cash, but that was something I hoped to never have to do).

"Would you like to see a nurse? She can check your vitals . . . triage. It's free."

Wonderful. What a lovely word. Free.

"Yes, let's start there." I smiled, relief flooding my veins. Finally, the kid was getting some medical attention, after two hours of driving in snow and clinic hopping. Antonio's next plan was a phone call to Brazil, at this hour disturbing his sleeping parents.

Now here's where things get interesting. As Antonio gingerly sat in the triage area, and I to his left, we surveyed the scene. There was an elderly man moaning in pain on a stretcher, a schizophrenic who I suspected hadn't taken meds in some time, and a kid with some kind of sporting injury. Add to this someone who was very clearly homeless, and another man who looked like he'd been recently released from some kind of correctional facility. Lastly, and my favorite, the drunk man who was gesticulating spasmodically. The whole thing was rather unpleasant, save the drunk man whom I found rather amusing (I'm not going to lie, I needed a laugh at this point). I moved closer to Antonio. After all, we were a team now, and frankly I didn't want the man who resembled a criminal swiping his wallet. We had enough to deal with. His credit card replaced once already, this wasn't happening again on my watch.

And then the questions started as the nurse checked his vitals. What had he eaten recently? Now here's the thing: Antonio had a fondness for McDonald's. And Pringles. I'd vacuum his room weekly and unearth enough empty Pringles tubs to fill the recycling bin twice over. Okay, maybe not twice, but there were a lot (and let's not forget that I was providing three homecooked meals a day). Now, on that particular afternoon, Antonio had indulged in something of a bread-and-butter bender (my former self could relate to that one). The reason I knew this is that when I'd left for work, the butter dish and bread bin were both full. Antonio had been the only one home early that day, and before leaving for the hospital I noticed that not only was two-thirds of the bread gone, so was the vast majority of the butter. Now granted, the butter was softened and easy to spread, as I preferred to keep mine in a butter dish on the kitchen bench. This went partway to explaining what happened next.

The good news was that Antonio did not require surgery, nor did he die that day. Essentially, he needed to poo. Heading home (the snow deeper still), we stopped at the pharmacy as the nurse had recommended a painkiller and something to help with his overloaded bowels. At this point I was on the phone with the other four to remotely organize the evening's meal. I had but one thought: *I need to hide the butter. Perhaps the freezer?* (I'd solve that problem later.)

So we headed off into the drugstore in search of tummy-related medications. No sooner had I turned around, and Antonio was gone. How could I have lost a six-foot Brazilian so fast? And where the hell was he?! Time to search the aisles. I just wanted to go home; it had been a rather long day, and I still had readings to complete for my own academic pursuits. And then I locate my dear Antonio . . . in the *chocolate* aisle! Did my student have a death wish?! This is the same boy who had been dying but an hour before.

Chocolate bars in hand, he explained, "I think I might save these for later, Jane."

"Yes, yes, I think that might be a very good idea." I shepherded him out of the junk food section as quickly as possible. Was he also an emotional eater?! Much like my former self, Antonio did seem to have a complicated relationship with food—the irony not lost on me.

The upshot of this story was that Antonio's parents severely cut his pocket money. Whether or not he wanted to hit McDonald's before eating my lovingly prepared meals was now irrelevant. He couldn't afford to. And that was the last time that Antonio needed the emergency department.

Only one other time did I manage to lose my charge, and this time, the terrain was slightly different. You see, Johann, my German student, was an excellent skier. My children and

I are also skiers, so off we went, one early morning—a day trip to Whistler always welcomed by all. Plus, Antonio was excited to learn. The (still shared) car loaded the night before, we set off in the dark in order to hit the mountain when the lifts opened.

Johann brought along a friend, a lovely young man (fellow German exchange student-mini-adult). It was 6:00 a.m., and I found myself passing back protein drink boxes, muffins made the night before, yogurts and so forth to the five hungry teens in the back. The atmosphere in the car was hectic but happy. It was still dark out and the road winding, skis safely stowed in the roof box. Concentrating hard, I was juggling as always. I was also acutely aware of the fact that, while driving, I held the lives of not only my own children, but of three more in my hands. It's really a monumental responsibility when you stop and think about it.

Johann told me later that his friend observed me and whispered in German, "Respect, man. I would not want to be Jane right now."

Well, he probably didn't want to be me later that day either. Having returned to the car at the end of the day at our agreed time, we found ourselves one man down. Antonio was missing. Now I should probably mention here that Whistler Blackcomb is the largest ski resort in North America, and by a considerable margin. There's no shortage of places to get lost outdoors. And you can probably see where this is going . . .

I tried Antonio's cell number. No answer.

"Oh no. Where do you think he is, Mummy?" asked a wide-eyed Alex.

"I don't know, darling." None of us did.

My German boys were giggling to themselves at this point, finding the whole situation quite amusing.

If these were the days of AirTags, I swear to God, I'd put a tracker on every kid in my care. Or in their backpacks. Now that would have helped. Well, except for the fact that I'd also have been tracking the tourist who now owns Antonio's lost backpack . . . but then we would have been able to find it! The mind boggles. (FYI: In 2024 I have an AirTag on everyone's shit. Brilliant invention.)

Finally, my cell rang.

"Ahh, Jane, I think I'm lost."

"Oh dear. Okay. We'll come to you. Don't move!" I instructed.

"Now take a look at your phone. Where are you?" God bless Google Maps and precise GPS locations.

Now at this point, we were at the bottom of Creekside, on the Whistler side of Whistler Backcomb.

"Ah, I'm on Blackcomb. I think I took a wrong turn down a run! I'm really sorry, Jane."

"Yes, yes, I think you might have. Don't worry. Just don't move." I was talking slowly and clearly at this point.

Of course, it's okay. He's safe and not injured, lying in a snowdrift somewhere. Life is good. The boys were, of course, still chuckling. We all knew that if someone was going to get lost, it was going to be my absent-minded professor of a student.

Alex was confused. "Why didn't he just read the signs, Mummy?"

That was a very good question, and I have no idea. After all, Antonio's English reading comprehension was excellent at this point.

So off we headed, retrieving my dear, hapless Brazilian boy.

"Ahh, Jane. There's a problem in the kitchen. . . . I think you'd better take a look."

Oh dear.

I was beginning to learn that any sentence out of Antonio's mouth that began with an apprehensive *ahh* was bound to bring news of misfortune. This morning proved no exception.

Let's begin with the time: 6:40 a.m.—too early for problems. Fortunately, we were long past formalities, as Antonio stood nervously at my bedroom door. *What on Earth had happened?* I wondered. I was about to find out as I reluctantly climbed out of bed and wandered down the hall in my pajamas.

"Ahh . . . I think it maybe got too hot and boiled dry?!"

"Yes, yes, I think it might have . . ."

I looked around, immediately thankful that no one was in the kitchen at the time. You see, Antonio's Bialetti stovetop espresso maker had exploded. Everywhere. Even the faded (now speckled) ceiling wasn't immune. The metal was in four parts on the floor. A chunk of plaster was missing from one wall, such was the pressure on impact. And microscopic coffee grounds were covering every surface of the tired cream kitchen. Not even the photos on the fridge were spared the impact.

Fuck me.

"Ahh, Jane . . . I have to get to class. I have early band practice!"

I smiled—an automatic response—concealed my frustration, and I heard myself say, "Of course. You've got to get to school. I'll clean this."

Antonio and I both sighed, for very different reasons at this point. The kitchen was a disaster.

Now this would have ordinarily been the end of it, only it wasn't. You see, several days later Antonio returned from a shopping expedition with . . . wait for it . . . a brand-new Bialetti! Not kidding.

"*Oh* no. No, no, no, no, no."

I was clear on this point really.

"Here's what we'll do, Antonio. I'm going to pack this away, and when you fly home in June, you can have this back to pack in your luggage, okay?" I was firm on this point. "We are not using this here. *Ever.*"

He looked surprised, bewildered, and just a little annoyed. Then again, he wasn't the one to clean the kitchen post-explosion. Of course, he was happy to roll the dice again. I, for one, preferred to err on the side of caution. I knew full well that my absent-minded charge was just as likely to get distracted and leave the kitchen again, resulting in another overheated, exploding Bialetti. Well, not on my watch.

Possibly the most ironic piece of this tale took place many months later. You see, I received a WhatsApp text from my dear Antonio in Brazil where he was living again with his parents and awaiting university classes. The message began with the following: "Jane, you were right . . ." (I certainly was this time.)

You see, Antonio had successfully blown up his second Bialetti, this time south of the equator. I should point out that our rental kitchen was never quite the same after our northern hemisphere explosion. I could only wonder as to the state of his parents' kitchen, as empathy for his parents filled my mind. *God help them, and let's hope they have a good housekeeper down there*, I mused.

Johann (mini-adult German student) called it, nailing my kids early on, with a wisdom that defied his age. "Cerulean is East Germany, Emily is West Germany, and Alexander is the Vatican. Kinda neutral, but still likes to mess with everyone!" And I still don't think anyone has better understood the dynamics and personalities of my three children so quickly.

At this stage my disordered eating still surfaced from time to time. While I maintained a pretty healthy weight, I wasn't immune to the stressors of day-to-day life—trips to the emergency department with my students during snowstorms and whatnot. And what was I hungry for? Looking back, adult conversation. And five minutes to myself. Privacy was limited in that rental house; my escape was the kitchen. After all, I was already spending most of my waking hours there, preparing food for an army of hungry teens. Comfort baking was that old familiar standby. Ahh . . . dysfunction. How easily I could slide back into your sweet, buttery embrace. Until I couldn't slide back into my jeans.

And then the pandemic hit. And I ate. Everyone ate. And everyone started baking. After all, we were all in the kitchen 24-7. I discovered intermittent fasting. Brilliant in theory if you don't then break your fast and devour everything in sight that you've restricted during the preceding fast. Something of a problem. Science tells us to avoid intermittent fasting if we have an eating disorder or are recovering from one. I didn't get the memo. Instead, I fasted. Or I tried weird combinations of restriction. I also walked. A lot. It was the one thing we could do during lockdown. It wasn't for a few years yet that I would truly make peace with my body. In the words of Geneen Roth, those were still the days of hungering.

youtube

Not until we are lost do we begin to understand ourselves.

—Henry David Thoreau

"Mummy, I identify as nonbinary!"

Cerulean announced this with wild, anxious enthusiasm as they marched downstairs and into the sunken lounge room. Charlotte and I looked up from our glasses of red wine in surprised bewilderment. Also recently divorced, my newest Vancouver friend had just dropped by after work, and just in time for what would be a defining moment in my child's life.

"That's great, honey!" At that point I really wasn't sure what else to say. Just shy of sixteen, Cerulean was far more aware than I of the enormity of this moment. That was four years ago. And no, it wasn't just a phase.

"She's just watched too much YouTube!" was Jan's initial response.

"No, mum, I don't think that's it. After all, I have three children. All of them watch YouTube, and only one of them identifies as nonbinary." Bless my loving mother. She really didn't understand. Born in 1954 and raised on a sheep farm in rural Australia, the poor woman had to google "nonbinary" to have any concrete idea of her grandchild's new identity. Not one to support gay marriage, my father's views are even more antiquated. He's yet to evolve to even the same degree as Gary Jeffries, fellow Aussie and father of comedian Jim Jeffries. While I fully support gay marriage, I'm inclined to agree with Gary Jeffries on the subject: "Well, I guess they deserve to be as miserable as the rest of us!"

Indeed.

As an ally and fierce advocate of the LGBTQ+ community, of course I agree. Absolutely. We should all have the right to be miserable, bound to another soul for eternity should we so choose. Why anyone would want to anymore, I have no idea, but I'll get to that later.

I was born in 1977, and I admit that when my child told me that they identify as nonbinary, I also had to consult google for a better understanding (but with more initial understanding than Mother, let's be clear). Having grown up in a white, conservative, comfortably racist outback community, well, good Lord, people weren't even allowed to be gay in 1985. Everything was taboo. And God forbid you were different. Mine was a rather sheltered childhood. I recall in my high school of seven hundred, there were only three people with skin that differed in color from my own: The boy of Asian descent (son of the town doctor) and two aboriginal students. Different just wasn't allowed, and my thunder thighs certainly weren't.

I knew that the road ahead for Cerulean wouldn't be an easy one. Thankfully we'd wound up residing in Vancouver, a generally tolerant and inclusive city. I also knew that Cerulean had inherited my determination and confidence to forge their own path, and to hell with the opinions of others. To this day, it serves them well.

My child had to go one step further of course. It wasn't enough to confound their grandparents with their rejection of gender; they also decided to adopt a vegan diet.

"Gender is a social construct!" they declared.

I don't dispute this.

"Animal agriculture is destroying our planet!"

I also won't dispute this. At this point in my life, we'd all learned *a lot* about cows. Their passion was honorable—if a little exhausting. Cerulean became obsessed with cow welfare. Naturally I saw the parallels in my own tendency toward obsessiveness. Apples and trees again . . .

I couldn't dispute Cerulean's arguments; they were correct on both points in my humble opinion. My mother, on the other hand, disputed both points—although she's now coming around on the second. Such was her distress at hearing that her eldest grandchild no longer ate meat, I think she came close to booking a flight and making the trek to British Columbia to cook Cerulean a steak. Raised on a farm, this decision was beyond my mother's comprehension. And make no mistake, for Cerulean, this decision was driven entirely by ethical, moral, and environmental imperatives. Formerly a voracious omnivore, I remain impressed by my eldest child's convictions.

Ever the optimist, I decided to embrace the challenges of plant-based eating. Thanks to the insanity that is the internet, millions of vegan recipes were available at a moment's notice—and access them I did! Throwing myself into this new challenge, we all learned quickly that plant-based eating is delicious. And it was also good for my perpetual diet. Everyone's waistlines benefitted. How could they not? Michael Pollan is right in his decree: "Eat food. Not too much. Mostly plants."

While not a vegan myself, to this day I aim for a plant-heavy intake. After all, plants are usually full of fiber. A good thing: I get full faster. We all do! Cravings are curbed, and I'm convinced that when we eat a ton and a variety of plants, our body is finally getting all of the vitamins and minerals that it needs (or a far closer approximation of this requirement). I'm also pretty sure that no one died an early death due to eating too much broccoli. I don't see a downside.

Now, despite heavy lobbying by Cerulean, my younger two children compromised and embraced a pescatarian diet. They weren't ready to give up salmon or Greek yogurt, and quite frankly, neither was I.

"I don't know of one student in this school more negatively affected by the pandemic than Cerulean," confided my child's school counselor. Now in a school of fifteen hundred students, this was no small statement. And he was right. For my exhausted neurodivergent child, the pandemic was the tipping point. My beautiful eldest child had been masking for too long, in an attempt to suppress and hide their autistic behaviors. Not surprisingly, autistic burnout was the end result. For too long, they had been trying in vain to fit into a neurotypical world, and their neurodivergent brain said, "Enough!" Now this is not my story to tell and would require another book, so I will attempt to keep this brief. Ultimately, a diagnosis was made late in the pandemic. My kid was autistic. Suddenly their world made sense. They made sense. And we got it. Everyone got it.

Prior to this diagnosis, these were very dark times. Brian and I were at a loss. For a kid already struggling with sensory overload, the fear of germs, the masks, the remote schooling without warning, well, it was just too much. Way too much. They took to bed, the weeks rolling into months. Showering become a weekly event, and that was on a good week. While heartbreaking to witness, I also found the feelings of my own helplessness overwhelming. I wanted desperately to fix my child and couldn't. The eventual realization that all I could do was love them unconditionally and provide support when they asked for help was oddly comforting.

I'm pleased to report that during these trying times, I neither became an alcoholic nor did I resume comfort eating (that was a minor miracle in itself, given the stress the entire family was under). I simply wasn't that same girl anymore. Of course, neither was my eldest.

tinder

If everything around you seems dark,
look again, you may be the light.

—Rumi

Despite having dear friends, hectic days, and living with five teenagers, there were periods of loneliness and a deep yearning for connection. Not to mention the physical intimacy that was missing at this point in my life. Frankly, I just needed to get laid. So what did I do? What many other newly single, separated people on the planet resort to nowadays. And with no idea of the madness that was to follow, I downloaded a dating app.

Tinder was horrific. And an overwhelming waste of time. Actually, most dating postdivorce was horrific. I'm convinced that there's a special place in hell reserved for men who ghost women via online dating apps—for that matter, any human who ghosts another online, irrespective of gender. And did I say men? My mistake! Men were in short supply. What Vancouver did seem to produce en masse was a plethora of boys, although that would be an insult to my son, who has more manners and sense of decency than the boys I met online. Tinder and Bumble were positively rife with overgrown boys.

I can't say I met a lot of men, and this experience alone constitutes another book. As a woman, if you've ever wanted to feel like crap about yourself, question your worth, obsess over your profile pictures, and generally experience a perpetual rollercoaster of excitement, anticipation, infatuation, disappointment, hurt, and pain, go ahead and download a dating app. Of course, free for the basic versions. Let's make these as accessible as possible for any pervert with a smartphone! In under five minutes some prick with a girlfriend/wife/whatever can have himself a fake online profile. He doesn't even need a friend to take the photo. Oh no, let's just throw a bathroom selfie online, because we all need to know where you relieved yourself before taking the blurry picture. Bonus points for a toilet in the background.

People seem to have no concern for, or appreciation of, the fact that ignoring communication from another human being with whom you've shared time is cruel. It's unbelievably rude and hurtful. What is wrong with people today?! Have they forgotten all sense of decency? Whether it's a shared walk, coffee, drinks, or bodily fluids, isn't a twenty-second "Nice to meet you, and I wish you well" text preferable to silence? Do these exchanges not warrant some form of polite communication in response? Is it necessary that online dating be devoid of all humanity? And full of assholes?!

It's probably not surprising to learn that we are hardwired to take the path of least resistance, and for the plethora of Tinder Swindlers who abound, this path is avoidance. Ghosting. It's incredibly easy. With little if any emotional investment after one or two dates, any uncomfortable texts are simply avoided entirely. Block, delete. It's the first course of action for many when any feelings of stress or anxiety arise. The problem is that it's also rude, cruel, and hurtful.

Are the men of Vancouver that lacking in a pair of balls (in addition to decency) that they are unable to send a "Thanks, but no thanks" text? It's not that hard. Perhaps it's a global phenomenon? After all, brief discussions with girlfriends in other cities and on other continents confirm that Canadian men don't have the monopoly on being assholes. It's far more widespread. God help us all. And as for the overgrown boys of Vancouver, I've concluded that they don't have a pair of balls between the lot of them.

I found the whole experience quite dehumanizing. Just a whole lot of boys running around behaving badly. Of course, I refer to heterosexual boys in search of women, and the exasperated women who sift through the time wasters in search of the very rare, elusive, yet still-to-be-found-on-occasion Good Man. Honestly, it was like looking for a unicorn underwater. Without oxygen. Now, I do appreciate that this was my subjective experience, and that many men have experienced similar disappointments and disrespectful treatment from women online. In fact, regardless of gender and sexual orientation, everyone I have spoken to reported stories of appalling rudeness. Why do dating apps bring out the worst in some people?

Boys behaving badly. I liken their experience online to being five years old again in a toy store, running around wildly, wide-eyed and overwhelmed. It's all so shiny and new and exciting! And so with reckless abandon and zero concern for any woman's feelings, overgrown boys will lie, charm, and fuck their way around the lower mainland of Vancouver. I doubt any other city on Earth is much different. One quite enthusiastic sex pest went so far as to send me a home movie. Oh no, no run-of-the-mill dick-pic for him.

Perhaps an amateur filmmaker? We can only guess, and I'd rather not. What I did learn on that memorable day is that some things you just can't unsee. What this amorous chap decided to do was film himself simultaneously masturbating while drinking beer and forward it on for my viewing pleasure. Or was it his? And was he trying to demonstrate his ability to multitask?! And who took the footage? And why, dear God, why?! The mind still boggles.

Block. Delete.

Thank you. Next.

"Oh, Jane, all men are perverts," Charlotte exclaimed, laughing.

"Yes, but these overgrown boys shouldn't be allowed access to technology. Whoever said it was dangerous in the wrong hands wasn't kidding."

Charlotte would join my students and I one night a week for a shared meal. I'd cook for seven (after all, what was one more?), and she'd bring the wine. Both single at the time, these were pleasant evenings, full of laughter and love. Where would we be as women without our girlfriends to help navigate the madness that is dating in our modern world?

Now, possibly the award for the biggest waster of my time goes to the man who so grossly misrepresented himself that I barely recognized him. If not for his wave and grinning face, I'd have walked straight past him. His online pictures were a good decade or more out of date, but that's not even the worst part. His photos gave the impression of some kind of personality. They lied.

I remember thinking to myself, before the first word was out of his mouth, *You're about to waste my time.*

And he did.

Thank you. Next.

Next was the enthusiastic suitor who felt the need to weigh me, literally. At the end of a rather pleasant walk and coffee date (to his credit, he insisted upon paying for my overpriced latte. You know the bar is low when this becomes a pleasant surprise). So, there we were, exchanging pleasantries when he abruptly put his arms around my waist and swung me into the sky at least two feet. Was I impressed with his strength? Well yes, after all, I'm not a petite, ninety-pound Asian woman (despite what Sally Newton said about my eyes). Was I baffled? Yes.

"I just wanted to make sure that I could pick you up!" was his enthusiastic explanation. Did I pass some kind of test? Feeling very much like I was about to be awarded a second-prize ribbon at the county fair, I bid him good day.

Another day, another horrific first date. The next one evidently fancied himself some kind of comedian—this one was also a good ten years older than his photos, I might add. So there he was with his beer, I with a glass of red (which, at this point, was doing nothing to make him look any more like his cute profile pic, circa 2000).

"I have a joke for you!" he exclaimed.

Terrific.

"Great, let's hear it!" I found myself saying. After all, I'm nothing if not a fan of comedy.

Now it will help to understand this joke with an awareness of the following: The itinerant young workers who keep the Whistler Blackcomb ski resort running year in and out are largely Australian. Now, knowing this, I will share his attempt at first date humor.

"Here it is!" he declared, looking over his second beer and asking, "Do you want to know why men can't get a blow job in Whistler?"

I stare. I think he was about to tell me.

"Because all the cocksuckers are in Australia!"

Laughing at his own joke for a good minute and a half, I looked on, bewildered, too tired to be disgusted. Did this man truly feel this was appropriate first date humor? Answer: yes. Was he also a probable sex pest? Also yes. And who uses the word *cocksucker* on a first date?!

I just can't believe I did my hair for this, I remember thinking.

Thank you. Next.

Dating shenanigans continued along the same vein until I'd quickly tire of the bullshit and delete the app, only to download it six months later and try again. Ever the optimist, I refused to give up. Not my style. I knew that I could grow old with ten cats, I just didn't want to. One or two, sure, but ten is a little ridiculous. Can you imagine the food bill? The kitty litter?! Anyway, I knew good men existed; I just didn't know where on Earth they hid. They certainly weren't busy drinking beer while masturbating, recording the experience for posterity, and sending the footage to strangers. Perhaps they actually had jobs? One did wonder in those early days.

Unfortunately, the horrors of online dating did nothing to help this recovering overeater. How easily my body insecurities were triggered. Certainly not helped the day one man-boy requested five full-length body shots before he would agree to meet in person for a drink. I had but one response for him: Fuck. Off.

Another shared the following wisdom on a first date: "Dating postdivorce is like searching through a used car lot for the best secondhand car!"

Where do men come up with this shit? Seriously?! Do they attend asshole school? How to be Rude and Thoughtless

101? I swear, I couldn't make this stuff up if I tried. How could anybody possibly think that this was appropriate conversation for a first date? I was continually horrified (and often offended) by the words and actions of these overgrown boys in Vancouver.

It wasn't easy remaining strong and confident with my body in those days. Of course, I was convinced that I just needed to lose five pounds. Five pounds until the man of my dreams would show up on my doorstep, flowers in hand.

Comparisons are dangerous. I'd find myself comparing my thighs with the thighs of other single women, and I'd always find myself lacking. Never quite slim enough for the Vancouver dating scene, and I later discovered why. Among women aged forty to forty-five, the North Shore of Vancouver has the dubious distinction of possessing the highest rate of eating disorders in the country. Judging from the women in the neighbourhood, anorexia and bulimia were at the forefront. Sadly, I was on the verge of becoming a statistic. After a particularly large meal with the children and another online rejection from a reject, I was in a very bad place. Bloated, hormonal, and terrified of returning to my former fat days, I threw up. In that ugly, dated blue rental house bathroom, I stuck my fingers down my throat and heaved until there was nothing left in my stomach. And then I leaned over the sink and cried.

Despite being extremely active and healthy by now, I felt I was never quite petite enough. A size 6 comparing myself to the size 0 and 2 figures of many of the women in my affluent neighborhood. There was a world of difference. Men would appraise me on a first date as a man appraises a prize steer at the county fair. And don't get me started on the hypocrisy. Grown men out of shape from years of boys' club-style drinking benders demanding unrealistic perfection from their dates. Why is it that a wealthy, successful man is allowed to grow old, bald, and round, while women are expected to have the body of a supermodel, the playfulness of a teenaged girl, the maturity and bank account of a successful career woman, and the demeanor and submissiveness of a 1950s housewife? How the fuck is this even possible?

And then it hit me. Fuck them all.

I don't need to be anything for anyone.

I woke up. I'd been perpetuating the stereotype, enabling these man-boys with my actions, quite unconsciously. Until I stopped trying. Never again would I throw up after a large meal. Fortunately, I was a failed bulimic. I couldn't stand the sensation, the taste, the bloodshot eyes afterward. I knew at my core that this wasn't the answer. I also knew that after years of actually throwing up due to anxiety, developing a binge-purge habit probably wasn't in my best interest.

So I started exercising intensely. Sometimes excessively. I was yet to learn to be gentle with my body. I took an inordinate number of walks. A heathier escape to be sure. I rarely escaped into the pantry these days, reasoning that a walk in the woods was far healthier. Despite the realization that I didn't need to look a certain way for any man, I still wished to look good for myself, to feel energetic, to feel comfort and ease in my own skin and in the clothing that I wore. Hence, I walked.

Now this chapter would not be complete without inclusion of the following Tinder Swindler story. A true swindler in every way, this particular online dating enthusiast was an actual criminal, and I learned of this in the most unfortunate way.

You see, this man and I had briefly dated, and unbeknownst to me, he was a functional alcoholic. Turns out he was also broke. And how did I know that he was broke? Because one evening while I slept, he slid out of bed and out the front door of my little rental home, taking with him my eldest child's credit card. That's right. This criminal *stole my child's credit card* while I slept.

Kept safely (or so I thought) in my purse, Cerulean's credit card then found itself on a journey that spanned several suburbs and liquor stores, and not with my underage eldest. Oh no! This Tinder criminal was cautious to only tap small amounts on each transaction, hence his multiple visits to several liquor stores over the following day. By the time I realized it, finding my purse one credit card down—and canceled the card—several hundreds of dollars had been (presumably) drunk. I didn't imagine he was saving the haul for his birthday. Further investigation revealed a bottle of red and a Costco-sized bottle of Tanqueray, both completely empty in my cupboard. Sadly, I realized that this boy (I can't in good conscience call him a man) must have been drinking while I slept. Did he take swigs of gin while I was in the bathroom?! The mind boggles.

This was by far the most horrific online dating experience of my life, and as I recall this now, I'm saddened. These dishonorable people also ruin online dating for the rest of us and for the good men out there who are sincere in their intentions. How challenging for them it must be to earn the trust of a good woman nowadays.

Hungry for intelligent conversation, I also ached to be held by a good, strong man. Kellie says that a hard man is good to find. Well, it turns out that a good man is also hard to find—damn near impossible. Most of the good ones were married. I did walk away with a dear friend courtesy of Tinder, and for that I will always be grateful. My beautiful friendship with Californian Brad began with one Tinder date and the following declaration: "An American and an Australian meet in Canada! What could possibly go wrong?!"

Four months later, the pandemic hit. And then the land border closed. And then we became friends. Somewhat of a serial dater, Brad's Bumble bunnies became so plentiful that a numerical system was required in order to remember them all. I'd seen this game played from the other side, you see. Brad (like many men I imagine) would use multiple dating apps concurrently, playing the daily game of Would I Fuck That? Simple, really. Men, being such visual creatures, bless them, take a mere nanosecond to swipe left or right. Yes or no. Details came later. Who is she? Who cares!

And this brings me to another dilemma with online dating: The illusion of choice. Of more. This never-ending supply of newly divorced and vulnerable single women, ripe for the picking. The logic is flawed. Realistically, of the endless matches, how many of these connections could possibly result in true love? That elusive chemistry? Shared values, hobbies, and interests? Not impossible, as I've learned, but bloody hard work. It's a numbers game requiring persistence, determination, and resilience. Not for the faint of heart.

Brad will concede that he is the most superficial man on the planet. He'll happily own this undesirable trait. The problem is, I think that many men are. In no way does Brad have the monopoly on superficiality. Are women the same? I'd argue no, not for the most part. Most women I've spoken to reveal that they require an emotional connection prior to physical intimacy. Most men seem to require a pulse (their own). Beyond that, who the hell knows?

"Mummy, what if he's a robber?!"

My young son turned to me, alarmed.

"Oh honey, he's definitely not a robber. Would I have a boyfriend who steals things?"

Alexander pondered this, eyes thoughtful, suspicious. "I guess not," he conceded, clearly not convinced. (Tinder Swindler Asshole Criminal aside . . . let's be clear.)

The enormity of this situation wasn't lost on me. My children were on the precipice of meeting my new post-separation-non-Tinder-pervert-hopefully-non-robber boyfriend. A kind man with three children of his own, plus his own brutal separation war story. We'd been stealing moments alone together for months. A gentle introduction made sense. Reserving judgment, my young son agreed to dinner together. I suspected it was his love of food that drove that decision, but either way, I was grateful.

The faded doorbell rang. How it still worked was beyond me in that falling-apart rental house, but I digress.

"Hi, come on in . . ." I almost whispered, smiling. The wise man before me bore gifts: three wrapped packages, plus flowers. Smart man. My children cautiously made their way downstairs. Unusual trepidation turned to excitement, their eyes widening. Emily gasped. Turns out my kids are easily bought. Then again, here stood a six-foot man with an actual grown-up job, carrying flowers. Perhaps so was I.

"Mummy, I don't think he's a robber anymore!" Alexander leaned over, whispering over his entrée.

"I'm glad, honey." Smiling again, I offered up a prayer of thanks and stifled a laugh. Not only did this new man turn out not to be a robber, stealing my son's coveted Lego sets, it turns out he added to the collection! For my ten-year-old son, life was good again.

How odd and how foreign it must have been for my three young children. Suddenly, a strange man was sitting at the dinner table next to their mother. My parents divorced once I was in college. Decades too late, but I was spared that new reality in my youth. Mind you, I would have welcomed a wonderful man and companion for my mother. Lord knows she deserved a good man, someone to take over the chopping of the firewood for once.

So there we were, my kids having to contend with the reality of their parents dating. How very surreal the whole thing must have been. Perhaps still is? After all, we consequence our children with this new reality, the result of parents unable to remain married.

I do believe that kids build resilience as a result of these challenges. A harsh lesson in the reality of adult relationships to be sure, but reality all the same. I don't believe in shielding children from the realities of life (within reason). If we sugarcoat and protect our children from everything, how will they ever cope with adversity when it inevitably hits them in their adult lives?

epiphany

*A wise woman once said, 'Fuck this shit,' and she
lived happily ever after.*

—Unknown

One earth-shattering realization came the day I concluded that I didn't need a man. Sure, I welcomed a boyfriend, provided he was the right one, but this epiphany changed everything.

Everything.

I no longer needed a man to feel complete, to *be* complete. None of us do! I know of many women who choose to remain in unhappy marriages for the financial security (and geographical stability for any offspring) that such a union provides. Well, financial security be damned! My goal was never to remarry. That's a hard pass. And if I'd wanted my financial security ensured, I would have stayed married. I just somehow knew that I'd be able to take care of myself and my children. I trusted in my abilities, my strength, and indeed the universe. On some very basic level, I just knew that I could get shit done.

I no longer sought in vain for external approval and acceptance from any man in my life. I no longer needed to search endlessly by swiping right on some dreadful dating app, and to be clear, they were mostly left swipes. I recall one man wearing a bacon suit in his profile picture. Yes, seriously (and no, it wasn't that amusing). A defining moment if ever there was one (my epiphany, not the bacon suit). Embracing my perfectly imperfect body and my fierce, unstoppable spirit, well, that changed everything. Once I stopped searching in vain for external love, approval, and acceptance of my thunder thighs, everything changed. Because I accepted myself.

Gone were the days of needing a boyfriend to feel complete. I was having way too much fun on my own anyway, so I sent the nice nonpervert on his way. I wasn't ready for the commitment that he sought. Enjoying adventures with my children, escapades with girlfriends, and fulfillment at work, it occurred to me that I actually didn't have a lot of time for a man in my life at this point. I felt strong, capable, whole. I still do. After all, there's just nothing as powerful as a woman who knows her own strength. Who said that?

Movement. An integral, welcome part of my days. I fell in love with hiking quickly and easily. Now a basic need, my therapy was among the old-growth redwoods and Lululemon. Inspired by Cheryl Strayed and her trek across a great chunk of North America, I decided to buy a backpack. With typical Jane enthusiasm that my friends have come to know well, I dove into overnight hiking the same way I dove into patchwork quilting, scrapbooking, mountain biking, and one thousand other hobbies. And now writing, I suppose. Not one to mess around, I began researching, hit the local outdoor store, and persuaded my reluctant teenagers that this would be fun. And yes—it is! (Persuading the children was helped by well-timed visits to their favorite bakery to gather energy for these mountain adventures, let's be clear.)

Now I have a theory about hiking, clearly growing in popularity. I'm convinced that, as a people, we are all hardwired to crave time outdoors for the simple reason that, since the dawn of time, we have lived outdoors. For the vast majority of human history, far more of our daily lives were lived outside. Only very recently have we all found ourselves subjected to fluorescent lighting, glaring iPhones, and the insanity that is reality television (an IQ test if ever there was one). And I would argue that none of it is in any way beneficial for the health of the human race.

And so, we hike. Ironically spending thousands on equipment to do so, we then pay $20 to secure a coveted overnight backcountry campsite and sleep on the ground. But oh, what a slumber! The billions of stars—portals into the great beyond—the ice-cold lakes for that early morning dopamine hit, and the blissful sounds of nature, both quiet and calming. Immersed in spectacular natural beauty, with nary the wail of a police siren, we recharge. No drunk revelers shouting or car horns blaring, and far away from the city commotion that has become my Vancouver reality, we escape now as a family. And such a healthy escape. Curiously, with my hunger satisfied in different ways, I often find my appetite quite low when hiking. Sure, the food tastes better outdoors, but even so I don't eat much. My soul being satiated, food becomes an afterthought.

Now, as you can probably imagine, I have been asked by those who know of my massive weight loss, "Just how did you do it?" Well, another turning point in shedding some serious pounds was hiking. Maintenance is bloody hard work, requiring blood, sweat, and tears, and hiking with my tribe always seems to ensure sweat, occasional blood loss, and intermittent tears. We now know that exercise helps crush anxiety and boosts mood, getting all those happy chemicals flowing. Dopamine and serotonin. Pretty sure I was missing these vital chemicals for a couple of decades . . . and then I found them among the old growth forests of British Columbia.

One of many favorite hikes, the Grouse Grind is mercifully close to my humble abode on the North Shore of Vancouver. Comprising 2,830 stairs, and an elevation climb of over 800 meters, this popular hiking trail is about 2.5 km in distance. It's also aptly named. Essentially, it's an 840-meter vertical set of stairs built into the side of the mountain that sits reassuringly to the north of North Vancouver.

I recall being convinced that I might become a statistic upon my inaugural hike. You see, at least once per year someone does die attempting this strenuous hike. I was hoping to evade death, and as I'm here to write this book, it's very clear that I did (despite the very unattractive sweating and foulmouthed swearing on the way up on my first ever hike—I was still some ways away from my current level of fitness at that point). I also wonder how accurate the reported number of stairs is, given that every year when maintenance is undertaken, more stairs are added to protect the fragile and exposed tree roots and soil below from erosion by a mass of outdoor enthusiasts.

To be fair, not everyone looks enthusiastic. Most amusing are the couples, you know the type. . . . You can just tell that one member of the couple has clearly coerced the other into this fun outdoor activity! By the halfway mark, neither looks thrilled, and someone is muttering Australian-style profanities. I confess to finding humor in their discord, another reminder of the benefits of remaining single. For me, hiking alone equals peace—my therapy time. And I don't have to deal with any man's shit, on or off the trail. Win-win.

The Grind attracts elite athletes, retirees, young families—pretty much everyone. It also attracts its fair share of ill-prepared Tourons (tourist-morons). I kid you not, after one early season snowfall, I took to the still-open Grind with enthusiasm and prepared with gloves, beanie (toque, for you Canadians), and metal spikes for my hiking boots. You get the picture—much like Dora the Explorer on a mission, I was prepared. Breathing audibly on my way up the first quarter, I came upon an alarming site. One young girl—wearing jeans, no less—was also sporting a pair of Ugg boots, the type that an Aussie would wear at home, indoors by the fire. This poor confused girl was attempting to climb a snow-covered mountain in Ugg boots. And as I left the parking lot, post-hike, I heard (before I saw) the ambulance that was making its way to the base of the mountain. To this day I wonder if it was Ugg-boot girl who slipped and fell.

enough

Stalking: When two people go for a long romantic walk together, but only one of them knows about it.

—Unknown

"I concluded that it was enough," shared Katherine. Not entirely fulfilled, a new friend in my new world was sharing her tale of marital woe. After deep reflection, Katherine decided that her sometimes unfulfilling long-term union was happy enough, and she made peace with her decision to settle. Sadly, her spouse didn't share her contentment; he announced rather abruptly one evening that he didn't love her, had never loved her, and was in fact in love with someone else. And of course, he was leaving. Sports car midlife crisis, packed bag, the whole nine yards. Devastation ensued, and sympathy and compassion were bestowed on her.

What I find very curious is that this same compassion isn't always extended to a woman who chooses to leave her husband, whatever the outward reason may be. Judgment and criticism were thinly veiled at times, and I found myself on the receiving end of some rather disapproving women. And I wonder, as there were only two people in my marriage, what on Earth made anybody feel that they had the right to an opinion as to my decision, my marriage? Did they live my life? Know of my inner heartache and angst? What gives another woman the right to judge? Do they feel betrayed? Jealous? Are they perhaps projecting their own unhappiness onto me? I do wonder if perhaps they resented my decision. A great many women are unhappily married and yet choose to stay put, deciding—much like Katherine—that it is enough. And no, it wasn't enough for me, and that remains no one's damn business but my own.

Perhaps they feel betrayed by one of their own? As a stay-at-home mother for many years, I belonged to a club, and unbeknownst to me, upon leaving my husband I had defied one of the core tenants of that club. I had dared to ask for more. I had dared to demand more. More for myself. Sacrilege! After all, who was I, as a married homemaker, to ask for more? To make that autonomous decision. Judgment was rife. And it hurt. One married friend immediately shunned me. You see, there are only two people in a marriage (typically), and there were certainly only two in mine; I was one of them. Everyone else would do well to remember that. And unless you are one of the two card-carrying members of any union, I implore you to keep your opinions to yourself.

Charlotte understood more than most. She, too, had made the very difficult decision to walk away from an unhappy marriage. The big house sold, the ex-husband angry, the need to go back to work nonnegotiable. Her young children would sob every Friday. That was change-over day, the crying for their mother as predictable as it was heartbreaking. Should Charlotte have stayed in a loveless union, living Thoreau's life of quiet desperation? I will fiercely debate anyone who answers that question with a yes.

Charlotte also had her share of dating woes—the perverts to contend with—before she met a kind, wonderful man. Her own real-life Tinder Swindler, Charlotte's dating history had the unfortunate distinction of requiring police intervention. You see, Charlotte had attracted herself a stalker. Now my dear friend, being stunning, lithe, and a little younger than I, is exactly the kind of woman who would attract a stalker on a dating app. She's gorgeous. Unfortunately, her stalker also thought so. Also unfortunate was the fact that he didn't seem to understand the word no. Despite not having a comprehensive grasp of the English language, he did excel at texting, and his tech skills were top tier. Unlike the assholes I met who failed to text at all, Charlotte's stalker was quite the opposite. He couldn't stop texting! After blocking him, her thwarted suitor decided that the only thing left to do was to book a flight and hop a plane. Much to her surprise one afternoon, this Toronto native and enthusiastic chap made his way to her front lawn, where he camped out, holding some kind of bizarre vigil until the men in blue mercifully intervened.

Good Lord.

To this day I'm thankful that I've never had a stalker. Well, not knowingly, anyway. If I have, he's done well to fly under the radar, unlike Mr. Toronto over here. Poor Charlotte was shaken for some time afterward, and as a single woman with two young girls, felt understandably unsafe in her home for months.

You know, I feel it only fair that I include a tale of a good man doing a good thing in this book—because good men exist, and they also do good deeds. I know. Yes, I was as shocked as you are. After all, I think one of the funniest bumper stickers I ever saw was in Australia (where else?) and it read: I Believe in Dragons, Good Men, and Other Such Fantasies.

Yes, I laughed too.

Of course, I was married to a good man, and I know that. As friends, Brian and I have an extremely amicable co-parenting relationship now—to the point of sharing Christmas dinners. My more recent disgust with men in general stems from my atrocious online dating experiences. How does anyone come out of that shitshow without PTSD—seriously?!

So anyway, here's how I know that good men exist (in addition to Brian). You see, one day I returned home to my humble rental house from another long, dull day working retail (in the post-separation, flat broke days), and I was greeted at the door by my non-Tinder pervert boyfriend holding a plunger.

Oh dear. Where my children are to be found, plungers are always a good idea. Seriously, what is it with kids and excessive toilet paper?! So there I was, removing my work coat, and my boyfriend declared, "Someone's a Super Pooper!"

The children descended into a fit of giggles. I was aghast. And here's the thing: The good man was *still smiling*, despite having just unblocked a toilet. Plus, he brought everyone takeout for dinner so that I didn't have to cook. Needless to say, my kids loved him. I loved him. After all, he made them laugh, fed them, and handled our plumbing mini-crisis (as opposed to running off into the night like the thief, never to be seen again), and if that's not proof that good men exist, then I don't know what is.

house

Wealth consists not in having great possessions,
but in having few wants.

—Epictetus

Space is a curious thing. Marriage in Australia meant a big house. Ridiculously big. My father-in-law would joke that walking from one end to the other required the carrying of water and a two-way radio, lest the intrepid traveler become lost along the way. And he wasn't far off in that estimate. Ironically, the children preferred to camp out on our monstrous master bedroom floor with their sleeping bags, night after night. After all, they were small at the time, and separation in their oversized bedrooms at the far end of the home made no sense to their little-child logic. Children need secure attachment, and banishment to faraway bedrooms did nothing to supply this need. We also soon learned—after building a monster home—that everyone, guests included, preferred to congregate in the main living/dining/kitchen space. Open plan, the style of the day, facilitated laughter, conversation, and intimacy. The remainder of the house was largely superfluous.

Australians have some of the largest homes on the planet. Our average single dwelling is quite enormous. Room upon room that is rarely utilized. It's ridiculous really, and I'm sorry to say that I contributed to the problem. Perhaps we need to obtain that which we desire, in order to figure out what we truly want. And it turns out that I would be entirely happy with a postage stamp-sized cottage, complete with my homemade quilts and a cat (maximum two). In fact, right now I am quite content with my compact apartment. Yes, more bedrooms would be welcomed by my growing teens, however with the Vancouver property market being what it is, a four-bedroom apartment would require selling many of my major organs on the black market to finance such a home. And realistically, I do still need these organs (and likely still wouldn't have enough cash). Sure, I could probably spare a kidney but that's not the wisest decision. After all, at forty-five. I'm hopeful of another forty-five years around the sun, should the gods allow this humble wish.

"Alex, get out of the Goddamn bathroom now!" is Emmy's regular refrain.

Yes, I've successfully taught my children to swear like sailors. Or Australians. Our apartment is cozy, however with a corner view over the mountains and city, it does allow a certain spaciousness of the mind, and I love it. If we had stayed in that excessively large home in Australia, I know full well that I would have less quality time with my kids. They would disappear into their own corners of the house, never to be seen again. A small home raises issues of privacy, no question; however it also forces connection, something sorely lacking today in our online world. I prefer the intimacy. My children are learning the hard way that cooperation and compromise are essential when sharing under one thousand square feet.

Of course, they can and do bounce back and forth to Brian's larger home, so no need to feel too sorry for them.

When they need the privacy of their own bedrooms, they can access that at Brian's. After all, 150 years ago, they would have been eight or ten siblings to a bedroom in some freezing hamlet in England. Their life is one of relative privilege, and if nothing else, I will have prepared them well for house sharing in their twenties.

My goal is to raise kind, resilient humans who contribute in society to the best of their abilities, and if I can succeed in achieving this, I will die happy. My baby girl and middle child, Emmy, is well on her way. There's only one small problem: As a budding pastry chef in the middle of her training, our home is now filled with baked treats of the highest order. Given my recovering eating disorder, I liken this to taking an alcoholic to a bar. Temptation is rife. Perhaps the gods are testing me? Despite this barrage of new temptation, I notice now that this food no longer holds the same power—inner fulfilment has neutralized these desires that were rarely born of physical hunger.

It's blessedly sunny out, and I need to get outside. The mountains beckon.

"Kids, Mummy is off to hike!" (Like many parents, I often refer to myself in third person. I'm still not sure why.)

"Okay, bye, Mummy!" An automatic response as their eyes don't look up from whatever TikTok is currently trending. At least they can't be pretending to do their homework; there's simply nowhere to hide in our small apartment. If nothing else, I will always know what my teens are up to, and I've decided that this is preferable to my former home of five thousand square feet complete with swimming pool. But I do miss that pool! It took decades to have the swimming pool of my childhood dreams, only to immediately realize that I didn't want the life that we had built.

What was I hungry for when I built that monstrous house? I didn't even know at the time, but I know now. When discussing the reasons behind the large home that we were constructing, my self-deprecating humor hid the shame of my excessive waistline. "Well, I'm not getting any smaller!" I'd declare to everyone as they inevitably commented on the size of our home.

Ironically, as soon as the home was built, we were to move again, that beautiful family home now a very distant memory.

"Let's sell. It's too big," I announced. The conversation prior to our next relocation. The first of many . . .

"We'll be in Canada. It's just a hassle!" I reasoned. My dream home had fast become a nightmare.

"Couldn't you have figured this out, Jane, before we built this?!" A fair question from my then-husband.

I had to build a huge house to realize that I neither needed, nor wanted, a huge house. And no, the irony wasn't lost on me either. You see, these monster homes need to be heated. And cooled. And cleaned. And it's a lot of bloody work! Not to mention that from an environmental standpoint, they're an ecological nightmare. Truly. Yes, we had three growing children, but that house was large enough to rehome several families of refugees. And another three children. Looking back, I was clearly filling a void. Hungry, and I didn't know what for. Thinking a huge house would bring happiness, I went right ahead and built it. Seeking fulfillment, I failed.

Postdivorce, the cats stayed with Brian. He had the space. I'd willingly given up quite a bit when you think about it. My privileged stay-at-home mother role. My kids half-time. The big house in Australia. The pool. My cats. My financial security. My share of the retirement savings. The price was high. But I did gain my freedom, and that remains priceless. Is there sadness when I think about the divorce now? Of course. Years on, I'm still aware that this is not the life that Brian asked for in his forties. He didn't sign up for life as a single father, and I pray that he finds happiness again. He deserves that. We all do.

gravity

Gravity is a plastic surgeon's best friend!
—My surgeon

T here is no pleasing anyone. First, you are too fat, eating too much! Everyone is concerned for your health, or so they say. . . .

"Jane, time to stop eating!"

"Jane, get out of the fridge!"

"Jane, you must be full!"

Post-weight loss provided a curious barrage of new comments . . .

"I hope you're eating enough, Jane!"

"Oh, you don't want to lose too much weight, Jane."

"Oh dear, you're starting to look unwell!"

"Jane, I'm worried about you. You're starting to look gaunt!"

"Oh, Jane, your face is losing its fullness. Oh dear."

Well, I did think that this was the point?! (Well, not the looking gaunt part, but you get the picture.)

Kellie was several months postpartum after her first child, and a little fuller-figured, when her uncle called her Chubba-Wubba Chipmunk Cheeks. Well, fuck me. Can you imagine? A grown man, referring to a woman and new mother in this way. Outrageous. Some people truly believe that they have the right to comment on another person's weight, the way we mention the weather of the day. How unbelievably offensive—and outrageous. It's completely impossible. The never-ending judgment! To this day, well-intentioned people who have known me a very long time will share their thoughts about my body. And I would like to know, when did my body become the subject of such scrutiny? And why? Doesn't anybody have a job to do? Something to otherwise occupy their thoughts?

No one tells you of the downsides of weight loss. The cost of buying new clothes, the loose skin, to name but two. A wonderful problem to have, with the first being a more economical fix than the second.

"Put a belt on!" was my ex-husband's ever practical advice.

Well, yes, I could put a belt on, Brian. But does that allow me to celebrate and honor my newly fit physique? Does it acknowledge the years of hard work, the endless workouts, rain or shine? No, it does not. Needing to buy new clothes was a wonderful problem to have.

As for gravity, well, that is no one's friend—I should know. The ravages of three pregnancies and subsequent breastfeeding (each baby for one year or more), plus the considerable weight loss left me with enough loose skin to donate to a burn unit at my local hospital. Plus, my formerly perky breasts had gone all *National Geographic*. It really wasn't ideal. Unfortunately, I attempted to diet the skin away, which I would later learn is impossible. You can diet away the fat underneath the skin, but not the skin itself. Sure, elasticity varies person to person, but evidently, I wasn't blessed with elastic skin any more than I was blessed with a happy, loving childhood full of summers at lakes and noodle salads. I wasn't dealt those cards.

And so, I stopped eating. I knew enough to know that I was again playing a very dangerous game, courting anorexia. Thankfully my voracious appetite prevented me from succeeding; I got hungry. I was a failed anorexic, and in hindsight, I can see why. I was exercising at that point in my life with the fervor of a religious zealot and had built considerable muscle. My metabolism was likely on fire, and my newly discovered muscles were demanding fuel, protein, and healthy carbs for energy. Still, I knew that I had to do something. A meeting with a wonderfully capable plastic surgeon followed.

"I have some patients who come to me and tell me that if they knew that their body would look like this after the weight loss, they wouldn't have lost the weight," he shared. Such is the discomfort of the extra skin, particularly in extreme cases. I can only imagine, knowing all too well what that postbaby tummy felt like. The cost of this surgery prohibitive, it would be years before I was able to return to my dear surgeon and green-light Operation Burn Unit.

Told I was a good candidate when I returned, as I had maintained the loss for many years at this point, my surgeon extended a kindness that I will never forget. The cost of this procedure had increased substantially, and with full awareness of my situation as a single mother (solo parent!) to three teenagers, the good doctor (and good man!) honored the quote that he had initially given me several years prior. I was both surprised and moved by this kindness.

My tummy was never going to recover without surgical intervention, and I was acutely aware that my plan to grow old with ten cats wasn't looking any more appealing. It was time for action. At this point I'd completed grad school and had earned a little money. I don't regret a cent that I spent on the surgery.

"You've done all the hard work, Jane. It's very impressive," he commented.

"Thank you! I'm definitely a work in progress!"

I smile, acutely aware of my lifelong healing journey. Personally, I found the lovely doctor rather impressive himself. Naturally, he was happily married with a beautiful wife.

I'm pleased to report that the end result was nothing less than phenomenal.

"Gravity is a plastic surgeon's best friend, Jane!"

Well, his scalpel was now mine. The man remains a God in my eyes, and I told him so. I gushed, entirely genuine in my praise of his work.

"Would you mind phoning my wife and telling her that?" he quipped.

I really would have at that point, such was my overwhelming joy. I sensed that my surgeon also truly enjoyed working with someone who had worked hard to lose weight. This was essentially reconstructive surgery, after all. I wasn't going in for a Brazilian butt lift (why, oh why) or cheek implants. Yes, that's a thing too. I just don't get it. I've spent the better part of the last decade trying to make my ass smaller. Why on Earth would someone pay to make theirs bigger?!

One glance around the waiting room revealed several young women who were clearly there to further sculpt their appearance into something resembling a reality television star. I'm still baffled—and who is watching this shit anyway? It's sad, really, as many of them were likely quite pretty to begin with, only to walk out resembling someone who might scare small children on a dark night. They sure as hell scared me.

Perhaps these women struggle with the same body dysmorphia that I also struggled with, post-weight loss. I realize that for many, these cosmetic procedures can boost self-confidence and self-esteem, and I fully respect an individual's right to choose to modify their appearance, should they wish to do so. On the other hand, it would be remiss of me not to note that body dysmorphic disorder is a very real psychiatric disorder, and those that suffer with this find that they are dissatisfied with clinically successful cosmetic procedures, and often begin a cycle of repeated surgeries and interventions in a quest for perceived perfection that never comes.

My experience was overwhelmingly positive, and I feel that it's important to mention that I did this for me. I knew that I would look and feel more confident in a swimsuit. Hell, more confident naked. I imagine that most women who have given birth to several babies will relate to this feeling. Pregnancy and childbirth wreak havoc on a woman's body, with or without additional weight gain and/or loss. The extra skin remaining on my stomach was, quite frankly, uncomfortable—particularly in the warmer months. My surgeon also discovered a small hernia that he repaired at the same time, likely caused during my third pregnancy.

Ultimately, I decided that if I did ever join a monastery, never again to lie with a man, I'd still be happier joining with my lovely reconstructed tummy. This procedure was nothing short of life-changing, and I'm unable to put a price on the benefits to my physical and mental health. And after all, life is expensive, but it still remains popular! (I'd like to note here that Brian finds this common refrain of mine less amusing than I do. Either way, it's as true as the day is long.)

fire

Lust without love is pleasure.

—Unknown

I 've always privately maintained that rules are for other people. Now this belief does come in handy at times, let me tell you. Having said that, it does remain imperative to know which rules one should and shouldn't break. In any event, the following period in my life left me safe in this knowledge. The scene is in an elevator. Of course it is.

"Hello, would you like some help with that?"

I heard a voice, deep—a delicious Spanish accent. I looked up, and the hottest building handyman I'd ever seen in my life met my gaze, playful. Already aware of his effect on women (without a doubt), he gave a half-smile.

"Sure, thank you," I responded with my signature warmth, aware that I was likely encouraging conversation.

"I'm Javier."

How lovely, I thought as I enjoyed the view, appreciative of this small act of chivalry as he proceeded to carry my recycling to the huge bins on the ground floor in the parkade of my building.

"Jane."

"Very nice to meet you, Jane."

Ahh, that accent. Why are accents always hotter than the alternative? And a hot man who was actually thoughtful enough to take time out of his busy workday to accompany me and carry my kids' crap to the recycling room? Who knew these rare men existed?!

His delicious chocolate-brown eyes appraised me . . . and then the elevator door opened, whisking me off to reality.

"Ciao."

Ciao, indeed . . .

Javier's playful eyes proceeded to stay with me the rest of that spring day.

Fast forward two weeks. Same elevator. Same garbage and recycling run. I should note here that my teens consume *a lot*. We produce enough recycling for a small army. How? I still don't know.

"Ahh, Jane. *Bonita!*" The door opened to reveal the lovely Javier smiling at me. Without asking, his perfectly chiseled arms reached out to take my overflowing recycling bin, his tense muscles perfectly on display under the fitted gray T-shirt. *Delicious. I could get used to this.* Realistically, the lovely Javier could have been saying anything to me at this point in Spanish. I didn't care. I've always been a sucker for the romance languages, particularly when spoken by a super hot man. Both were to be my undoing.

It's at this point in the elevator that I had an idea. Ever practical, I'd recently succumbed and purchased a television. I'd refused up until this point, maintaining the view that my teenagers had more than enough screen time already, what with their TikToking and Instascrolling. The last thing we needed was another glaring, distracting piece of tech that would prevent them from going outside. Vitamin D deficiency anyone? But I digress.

"I was wondering, would you possibly be able to put my new television on the wall in my apartment? I'll pay you for your time of course! You see, I have the bracket but no drill . . . I'll call a handyman if you can't, no worries! I appreciate that you're probably very busy in this building . . ." Realizing that I was rambling at this point, picturing the young Javier in my bedroom (which was to be the location of the television), I paused, smiling sweetly. The elevator dinged.

I don't like a television in the lounge room; it distracts from conversation. As I lived alone half the time, I reasoned that I'd rather Netflix and chill from the comfort of my bedroom on a Friday night. Always preferable to some dreadful Tinder-pervert first date anyway.

"Yes. I can do that," his reply in English still a little stilted. Back to reality.

"Awesome, thank you!"

"What is your number? I will put it into my phone!"

Ahh . . . There was the accent again. Liking this plan more and more by the second, hasty arrangements were made. Javier was to come by after work on Friday.

I heard a knock. No need to ring the buzzer—the lovely Javier had access to every floor due to the restoration work that his company was currently completing within the building. In hindsight, it was all just far too convenient. Tool kit in hand, Javier and his warm brown eyes were smiling at me from my front door. Shoes came off, respectful as he unlaced his work boots.

"I don't want to make your floors dirty!"

Bonus points.

Walking into the kitchen, he noticed my recently poured glass of red. It was a Friday evening after all, and it'd been a long week of dealing with my children, my ex, supporting my friends and their challenges. Essentially everyone else's crap. Time to kick back. Now, at this point in the proceedings, I realized that I'm on the verge of playing with fire. Contemplating . . . my heart skipped a beat as I casually offered him a glass of wine, appraising this man who is essentially a stranger. After all, he's been working hard all week, hasn't he? And to his credit he did show up with supplies, in addition to his tool kit: Wall things that he had just driven to the hardware store to purchase for the task ahead after work, plus his drill. More bonus points. I figured the lovely young Javier needed rewarding. He didn't skip a beat. With warm eyes fixed on mine, he smiled and said, "Thank you."

I pour the wine as impure thoughts flood my mind. Or are they pure?

You may not be surprised to learn that the television didn't make it onto the wall that evening. Or the next. I was child-free that week; my apartment rapidly transformed into a Spanish love shack.

I maintain that there's not a woman over thirty who doesn't know of the benefits of candlelight (for that matter, is harsh lighting anyone's friend?!). Now this knowledge was to come in handy at this point in my life, and left me wondering, *Why did we ever make the switch to incandescent bulbs? Ever?! They flatter no one.* But I digress, again.

"Oh my God. It's like a porn scene with the handyman and bored housewife! Your life is like a porno!" This was Madeline's take on my current entanglement. I should mention right here that Madeline is, much like Sensible Susan, prone to practical, grown-up decisions. I, on the other hand, was tired of being a grown-up 24-7. It's exhausting. I had to adult daily, carrying the weight of everyone who needed me. Javier was the only person with zero demands. He didn't need me to carry anything for him. It was as close to perfect as a tryst with a hot Spanish handyman can be. And much to my delight, not only did he not need me to carry anything for him, emotional or otherwise, he could carry me! (And that's no small feat.) God bless his physical job and regular gym workouts. Let's be clear, his arms were chiselled to perfection. I melted. My Spanish paramour proved a surprisingly thoughtful lover, and with Javier I could play, devoid of responsibilities, his sweet Spanish kisses both endless and intoxicating.

"Well, you know what they say, Jane. You're only as old as the man you feel!"

Kellie was right. And that summer I was thirty-two.

Javier, I quickly realized, had no idea that I was in my mid-forties or the mother of three almost-grown teens. To this day I suspect he is still trying to guess my age and knew better than to ask. Smart man. Despite the weight gain and loss, I am blessed to look reasonably youthful. I seem to have that girl-next-door look that some men can't resist. Javier had no idea that day in the elevator that I was forty-four, and who was I to overshare?!

Javier, my five seconds of summer . . . gone when the leaves started to turn, and no doubt off to some pretty young thing. After all, he revealed in confidence that he did wish to start a family and settle down. Well, good luck with that. He's got a fifty-fifty chance of succeeding at that endeavor, and I truly wish him every happiness. He will no doubt make beautiful Spanish babies with a more suitable senorita than I. My baby-making days were over long, long ago. (I feel the need to mention here that the television did eventually make it to the wall.)

Ahh . . . How I do appreciate Latin men and their hot red blood.

My observant teens did eventually learn of my not-so-discreet liaison. You see, there was a fire alarm one day in our building, and out we all filed, at this point not knowing if this was an actual emergency. Now not being one to gamble with real fire, we all exited sensibly down the stairwell. And of course, who should be outside but the hottest foreman on Earth, who was at this point working in our building. Just what were he and his crew doing? Painting? Rendering? I'm still not sure. In any event, there we are, all milling about on the street in front of our home, speculating the cause of this alarm (burnt toast on the fifth floor, I was later to learn). So, I was outside with two of my teens, and he looked over, giving me that delicious half-smile and the slight tilt of the head, the subtle nod of *Hey, what's up, bonita*?

Trying to hide a smile, my ever-observant Emily catches me.

"Who *is* that Mummy?! He's very cute!"

Yes, yes, he is, Emmy.

"Is he the one who put up our TV?"

More questions. After all, the lovely Javier had left his drill in the apartment, and that one had taken some explaining on my part. My kids weren't born yesterday, and they were well aware that I was dating postdivorce.

"He looks very young!" she proclaimed. Did I detect a hint of disapproval? Perhaps surprise?

"Hmm?" I murmur.

Men really do have their uses at times, my mind thought, wandering. The whole scene that morning was very distracting really. We had the hot Javier to my right, and to the left, several ripped, lovely fireman were, at that very moment, running into our potentially burning building to investigate the cause of the alarm. It was all a little much to take really. And what is it about a fireman in uniform that is so irresistible?! Is it the element of danger? The inherent risk? The physique?

"Oh, Jane, he looks like trouble. Fun and trouble, all rolled into one!" This was Isabelle's take on seeing his picture.

"Fun is fun!" This rather astute observation from my Latin lover. Yes, yes, it is, Javier.

And that's exactly what he was that summer. And exactly what I needed. No longer needing external approval, or anyone to fulfill an inner void, what I needed was to get laid, nothing more.

Ahh, boys . . . men . . . So many boys; so few men. My mind wanders as I type this. The rain drizzles outside, early autumn and the coffee house is cozy, the latte warming. Latin music fills the air; the perfect accompaniment to the Latin lovers who fill my head with wicked, impure thoughts. Or again, are they pure? Desire, my kryptonite. I know you well. After all, as the brilliant Kurt Vonnegut advises us, "Make love when you can. It's good for you." And who am I to argue with that?

Months later I saw Javier, our paths colliding yet again.

"Hey, you . . . I had a feeling I'd run into you today."

Hmm. Really? And why do these charming men always, *always,* know exactly what to say?

"I've been thinking about you. *A lot.*" His eyes were heavy with meaning. "How you doing, *bonita*?" Head slightly bent, eyes playful as always. Oddly, he'd crossed my mind earlier that day too. Quantum entanglement indeed.

"Let's have wine!" Javier declared, smiling. "I will cook for you . . ."

A tempting offer, I declined. I suggested coffee, reasoning that I was far less likely to get into trouble with caffeine.

Of course, with an almost comforting predictability, the lovely Javier would intermittently drunk text. I'd awake naturally on a Sunday at 4:00 a.m. or 5:00 a.m. (thank you, perimenopause) to be greeted by some semidrunk, waffling declaration that he'd sent two hours prior. And no, the irony of this wasn't lost on me either. Just as I'd be awaking to begin my day, Javier would be rolling into bed with whomever he'd found to keep him warm the night before, after his drunk text to the Australian failed. I just can't do 2:00 a.m. anymore. Can anyone over the age of forty?! And I don't want to be awake at 2:00 a.m., listening to *doof-doof* music in some club that's cool for five minutes. I think I'm officially old.

The months rolled into years, and Sebastian would also intermittently reach out. Were his texts boredom? Desire? Had he exhausted his supply of fuckable women in the Lower Mainland that month? Possibly all three. I stayed away. Lessons learned too late, but like a child that eventually learns not to touch a hot stove, I avoided further injury. The past finally in the past.

The thing was, I was tired of dating. The merry-go-round of underwhelming first dates. It was time to take action . . . so I decided to manifest! Yes, seriously. I actually did. Having recently learned more on the subject and having a decent amount of confidence in my abilities at this point, I figured

I'd ask the universe for exactly what I wanted. So out to my balcony I went one late autumn evening, palms outstretched, staring up to the night sky. I allowed myself to surrender to the energy of the universe, trusting. And after thanking the universe for my many blessings, I humbly asked for a good man to be sent my way.

Please send me a wonderful, good man that I can share my world with.

And three weeks later, I met Dr. A.

dr. a

I am convinced that God does not play dice.

—Einstein

"Jane, are you sure he's a doctor?"

Brad's first question. This was the age of Bumble, so the question was reasonably fair.

"Yes, yes, I've already googled him. No red flags. Story checks out, so far."

"He just sounds too good to be true..." Madeline's concern. "There must be something wrong with him!" she declared.

"Well, I imagine I'll find that out in time," I reassured my responsible friend. After all, we're all imperfect, and I'm no exception. I had no illusions about the reality of this knowledge. I also maintained the 1 percent rule: In my experience, 99 percent of online dating enthusiasts are time wasters of monumental proportions, leaving the 1 percent who are genuinely seeking something real. After all, I was online, so I reasoned that there surely must be a few good men out there somewhere with whom I shared this common goal. As I was yet to stumble across a unicorn, perhaps I'd actually found that elusive, rare creature—the good man.

"I'm just worried that a month from now they'll find your body in the desert somewhere in Utah! Just be careful ... that's all."

"Of course," I replied. Madeline's continued caution was still very much ringing in my ears as I boarded a flight headed for Dr. A and south of the forty-ninth parallel, that invisible line that divides the Great White North from our southern neighbors in the States.

Wise advice. Having agreed to a sprinter-van-mountain-biking road trip to a remote locale, this wasn't an altogether unreasonable fear of Madeline's. After all, there are very real dangers for women who participate in the madness that is online dating, and I'd rather my life not end the way it started, in some godforsaken desert in the middle of nowhere.

Never being prone to caution, of course I jumped into our desert adventure much like I jumped into my homemade pool all those years ago. Ironically both resulted in mild illness. Now it turns out that the desert of Utah is much like the desert home of my youth—dusty. And much like the climate of my childhood, I succumbed to spring allergies, with a blocked nose that would have been impressive if it wasn't such poor timing. Hardly romantic, I sniffed and blew my way through many a box of tissues on that inaugural road trip, bringing to mind the unfortunate sneezing incident of my youth. Fortunately, Dr. A was spared the same fate.

"Here, take this," he instructed after rummaging through his medical kit.

"What is it?" Not being a huge fan of medication, I was equal parts suspicious and curious.

"It will help."

"Hmm . . . okay." Too unwell at that point to argue, I did as instructed. After all, he was the doctor.

Again, another benefit of dating the doctor quickly became apparent when I ingested the tablet that seemed to magically eliminate my headache, reduce the congestion, and provide some kind of mild high. Following that, it put me to sleep. Win-win. To this day I have no idea what the good doctor fed me, but I do remain grateful. It's probably best to point out that Dr. A and I had spent several days together prior to my agreeing to our van expedition. I would never advocate a trip with a complete stranger met on a dating app—I'm not quite that reckless! After all, as a mother to three children, I'm always cognizant of the fact that they need me alive, and I sure as hell don't want to leave them motherless.

It's hardly coincidence that at the very moment I realized I was already complete, whole, and happy without a man (can you imagine?!), I met Dr. A. Originally a farm boy from Nebraska, Dr. A and I bonded quickly over our shared experience of small-town life as children and our mutual love of the outdoors. Of course, I had reached that beautiful place in life where I was truly at peace and happily alone, content with my own company, and that of my dear friends and children. Perhaps the universe sensed this energy shift? Perhaps Dr. A did? Not to mention my powers of manifestation. Seriously, that shit works, and I now practice manifesting daily. (Yes, really.)

Now the good Dr. A may have also sensed this energy, this calm confidence that I radiated at the age of forty-five. What he was yet to understand was the nature of my profanity, and the intent behind it. Dr. A quickly learned that Australians tend to swear—we swear like sailors really, quite often, and I'm no exception.

What he professes to being confused by is the meaning behind the expletive. You see, our inaugural van trip involved a lot of biking. Being new to mountain biking, this also resulted in a lot of falling—me, not him, to be clear.

Essentially, my DNA is now scattered all over Utah. Seriously, if I had been murdered in the desert, I'm pretty sure my body would have been found. Like Hansel and Gretel dropping crumbs, I left a calling card of blood and skin from scrapes against rocks that were so bad they required the use of the medical kit again (that thing really was the MVP on our road trip).

By the time we got to Moab, after winding our way down south through Wyoming to Utah, I was bandaged up and down one arm and leg like I'd recently returned from war. But here's the thing: As I was falling off this mountain bike pretty consistently, there was swearing, and a lot of it. The problem was that Dr. A had trouble distinguishing the Australian frustration profanity from the rather more intimate, passion-filled "oh fuck." Quite befuddling to my American paramour. We'd be trying to maneuver all manner of body parts, attempting to mess around in the back of his recreational vehicle, and he could never quite figure out if my "oh fuck" was a good or a bad "oh fuck." As I'd managed to confound a man with a doctorate and Ph.D., I was secretly amused by the whole thing.

Back at home, I came swiftly to a conclusion about the next chapter of my life.

"I'm going to write a book!" I announced to Charlotte on one of our many morning walks.

"Well, you've certainly got plenty of things to write about," was her pragmatic response.

As the years had passed, we gradually exchanged our wine evenings for morning walks, to my benefit. Charlotte remains one of those fortunate creatures who can both drink wine and fit into her pants. Perhaps she was a missionary in a former life? She must have done something good because she was certainly blessed in this one.

"Well, Jane, you've certainly done everything that you said you would," was the initial response of Georgia, my best friend from Vancouver, to my literary declaration. And she's not wrong. I say with pride and all humility that when I make up my mind to do something, it's done. "Freight Train Jane," Brian once called me. "Impossible to stop." In hindsight, I tend to see this as a compliment. After all, a freight train will get things from A to B with reasonable efficiency. And much like myself, shit gets done.

I knew that I had to write this book. I needed to make peace with my past, make peace with the old Jane that I'd kept hidden in the box under the bed where the dusty, decades-old photos lived.

And why am I still so ashamed to admit that I used to be overweight (obese, according to my BMI)? Why does it hurt to write these facts? I know why. Because society told me that being fat made me unacceptable, unlovable, unworthy. A glutton. Lacking in willpower. Lazy. Greedy. Slovenly. It was never-ending.

And was I those things? Honestly, no. What I was, was overwhelmed. Exhausted. Anxious. Sometimes melancholy. And in need of respite, nurturing, and compassion. And here's the thing: The world wouldn't provide that. I needed to begin by extending nurturing and compassion to myself. No one was coming to save me. I needed to save myself.

moderation

We have nothing to lose and a world to see.

—Rainie Navarro

We all have the power of choice, that dizziness of freedom of which Kierkegaard speaks. We are blessed with the ability to choose. Sure, cards are dealt out at birth, and yes, I was born into a safe, democratic paradise (lead dust notwithstanding). And to be clear, I didn't want the cards at birth that I'd been dealt. I wanted Bella's cards, with two loving parents, a backyard swimming pool, and a father who went to work and came home and didn't shout. My father was depressed, sometimes not working for months at a time. For my long-suffering mother, she found herself in the unfortunate position of both sole homemaker and breadwinner; my father, too depressed to assume either role. But here's the thing—I wouldn't change my childhood. I had to live my life to become the woman that I am today.

Perhaps we are all born into the families that we are meant to have, in order to grow, to learn certain lessons, and evolve. To become the people that we are meant to be. We are born whole and complete, and it seems to me that my journey thus far, from my teens until now, has been a journey back home. One of finding that unbroken, carefree child who didn't yet learn to associate food with love—a poor man's substitute if ever there was one.

As I navigated my new world as a solo parent, grad student, and homestay mother to international students, I came to realize that we humans *always* have the power of choice. Always. Sure, at times the choice may be between two crap options, and I'll choose the lesser of the two, but nevertheless, we can choose! Some of us are dealt shit hands at birth—frankly mine wasn't the best, but it sure as hell could have been worse. So much worse. I consider myself one of the lucky souls who just happened to be born into a safe, free utopia such as Australia. I'm saddened (and sometimes frustrated) by the people who don't realize that we all have the power to play the cards that we are dealt at birth. Kenny Rogers was right; every hand's a winner, and every hand's loser, and I sure as hell knew that I was going to play.

I lost a client to an overdose, the news of his passing received while I was in Greece. His ninth OD. Much like a cat, it seems my client was also to have nine lives, and that day, my client was all out of luck. He'd survived the eighth while I was preparing for my first European holiday in many years, taking some much-needed time away from my rewarding yet intense new career. For the first time, I had a few dollars in my bank account and a voracious hunger to explore the world.

Staring up at the Arch of Apollo on the island of Naxos, one word came to mind: moderation. Apollo was known for—among a great number of traits—a fondness for moderation in all things. The irony of my client's overdose wasn't lost on me. Nothing about that lethal dose of fentanyl was moderate.

Moderation. Greece allowed me to refine this concept. As I stood there pondering my late client and the ancient Greek gods, I was drawn to the parallels in my own life, this ongoing journey of learning moderation in all things. Food. Exercise. Desire. Rest. Sleep. The art of balance; energy in, energy out.

The weather that summer was anything but moderate. The climate was angry, southern Europe under another intense heatwave thanks to our reckless abuse of the planet.

"*Mummmmmmmmmmmyyyyyy!* I've got cankles!" shouted Emily at the base of the Parthenon. Too many hours in the sun combined with too much walking (according to the children)—time for rest, shade, and some iced lattes. After recovering, we'd wander, awestruck, delighting in ancient monuments. Every cobbled path dependably led from one delight to another. The food was a continued source of wonder, at times a spiritual experience in itself. Sheep's-milk feta and herbed zucchini, spanakopita, Greek wines, the local cheeses, and olives fit for the gods. How I wished to bring these home in my carry-on! And perhaps a lovely Greek man, just for good measure. After all, who knew when I'd need help with another DIY project?!

Most amusing of all in Greece were the gift shops. Now I've been into far more gift shops on my travels than I care to admit. They're largely filled with the same repetitive paraphernalia: keyrings, fridge magnets, and poor-quality T-shirts that few of us want or need—and even less, look good in. I have to say that the gift shops in Athens are my favorite for two reasons. First, they sold some very lovely olive wood utensils and cutlery that I use to this day (and who doesn't love a practical souvenir?). The second was for the massive, brightly painted wooden penis bottle openers. Practical and obscene. Brilliant. The children were beside themselves. So of course, I had to purchase one to mail to Kellie. To this day she assures me that it's the gift that keeps on giving. Her kids amuse themselves by waving the giant phallus at houseguests, and her husband can open his beer. Win-win.

Amusing pranks aside, I can't help but reflect on this once-powerful ancient civilization. A few centuries of greatness, and they're reduced to selling dicks in the street. I should point out that while fond of Apollo, another god to give me pause was Dionysus, god of wine and pleasure. The youngest of the twelve who inhabited Mount Olympus, ironically Dionysus represents the complete opposite of Apollo—excess, revelry, and euphoria. Now the Greeks believe that any great festivity was made possible by this youngest god, and who was I to argue with them? And did Apollo attend these festivities? Did his view of moderation include the occasional celebration? Evidently, yes. Moderation in all things, including moderation!

Perhaps Dionysus represents a cautionary tale? After all, I know all too well what excess looks like, my former fat pants a testament to this lack of moderation.

Widely considered the most handsome of the twelve gods, Apollo was also a known chaser of mortal women. I would have no doubt fallen for his charms—being unable to resist a handsome womanizer seems to be one of my weaknesses (the other two being homemade cheesecake and online shopping for Reformation dresses). Known for his love of drinking, dancing, and singing, it was the Temple of

Apollo at Delphi that I was most taken with. It's hard not to be intrigued with the god of prophecy, sun, and light, among other things. Mind you, Cerulean just announced, "Mummy, did you know that Dionysus was also the god of phallus and fertility?" I did not. They really are a busy bunch. If Zeus was the god of thunder, what did this make Dionysus? God of Tinder?

We had the good fortune to visit the ancient ruins of Delphi on this holiday, and while I wouldn't wish to have the powers of prophecy, I did feel some very real energy at this sacred ancient site. Sadly, we were a few thousand years too late to meet with the Oracle of Delphi, but this was likely for the best. If I could know the future, I'd politely decline. I don't think it's ever a good idea to know what the fates have in store for us. What I did feel strongly while we wandered among the ancient ruins and stray cats was a calm certainty that I was meant to embrace Apollo's view of moderation in all things. I continue to work on this.

The children, on the other hand, were content embracing the multitude of stray cats that called Delphi home. Georgia, who accompanied us on the trip, ever fearful of germs, would sanitize everyone's hands after every interaction. (We went through *a lot* of Purell on this trip.) Naturally, the children wanted to smuggle one of the felines home in one of their carry-ons. The compromise was the purchase of dry cat food. We spent the remainder of the trip feeding these cats at regular intervals, island hopping with kibble and hand sanitizer. Both flowed like Dionysus wine, much to the delight of the local felines.

Our presence in Greece revealed to me something of a fork in the road: on one hand was the path of sex, drunkenness, debauchery, materialism, and ego—a feature of modern life. The other path was an entreaty to "know thyself," with the ultimate goal of discovering my true essence—that I'm so much more than my physical form. Yes, I was elated to feel confident in Greece in a swimsuit, thanks to my recent tummy tuck; however, did my physical form define me? My self-worth? Was I in danger of letting this be the case? I found myself sitting with some very difficult questions. After all, I was judged mercilessly when I was obese. And now I found myself being judged in a positive light. Society approved of my bikini body. I was deemed acceptable. How is this possibly okay? And did this change my inherent worth as a human—my spirit, my desire to be kind and do good? To strive to be the best mother that I could be (and losing my shit less often in the process)?

A monumental "aha!" moment occurred. Yes, I was thrilled to be truly comfortable in my own body, able to sit with ease and wear a pair of pants that, for the first time in decades, would actually fit properly, but none of that mattered if I allowed myself to attach my self-worth to my new external form. Because we must never let our external form define us or allow ourselves to judge another based upon their physical appearance. The only thing that matters is love, kindness, fierce compassion, and remembering every day of our lives to wake up and attempt not to be an asshole.

Now on another note, I learned in Greece that sleep is absolutely essential for cognitive function, and far more important than most of us realize. I certainly realized it when I lay awake, staring at the mustard yellow ceiling of our Airbnb at 3:00 a.m. in Athens. Unable to sleep in my economy seat (how people do is still beyond me), I struggled to recall any of this new language in the first forty-eight hours—it really was all Greek to me. Matthew Walker, in his seminal work, *Why We Sleep*, tells us that without adequate rest, new knowledge learned in the daytime is unable to be shifted into longer-term memory within the brain, to be used for retrieval at a later date. As it was, my traveling party—consisting of Emily, Alex, Georgia, and her two children—became perplexed at my lack of retention. How could I still not remember "thank you" on the second day? Well, I knew how. I couldn't sleep! Then again, I did grow up surrounded by lead dust. Perhaps this went a little way to explaining my difficulty in learning a new language in my forties.

This limited grasp of even basic Greek did prove problematic, as time and time again people would look at Georgia and me, together with our four teenagers, and assumptions would be made. Now while it didn't bother me that some assumed that we were partners, I did try and explain "No, no . . . we're just friends!" After all, what if some delicious Greek god of a man was in the vicinity and caught my eye? Well, between the four teenagers and my female traveling companion, I was in no danger of being propositioned by any man, Greek or otherwise.

"Big family!" one elderly gentleman exclaimed, taking one look at us all.

Sighing, Georgia responded, too tired to protest or attempt to explain again, "Yes, yes . . . *big* family."

We gave up. After all, what did it matter? Mind you, when Georgia lost her makeup bag midway through the trip, she was less than thrilled. "Great! Now everyone will think that I'm the butch one!" huffed a frustrated Georgia.

Attempting not to laugh at this, I failed. She made an excellent point.

Greece was magical, and I long to return. For the people of this country, their cup really does appear to runneth over, much like Dionysus and his never-ending cup of wine. While still enjoying a tipple with lunch and dinner, some Greeks manage to live longer than most other people on the planet. Five blue zones have been identified on Earth, regions where populations are found to live the longest, and more importantly, the healthiest lives. Unsurprisingly, Ikaria, a small Greek Island makes the list. Of course, if Greece is a blue zone, Broken Hill must surely be a red zone—one huge lead-dust-polluted red flag.

While visiting the Peloponnese region of Greece, we witnessed this life-prolonging culture firsthand. While not Ikaria, the lifestyle seems similar enough to safely draw conclusions (informally, anyway). A plant-heavy diet; consistent, moderate physical activity; and social engagement are all identified as contributing factors in this longevity.

People with the good fortune to inhabit one of these blue zones will likely live up to a decade longer than the rest of us. And not just longer, but also happier lives from all accounts. They remain active, vibrant, and productive until the end. Now witnessing this—the wine, the cheese, and the happy old people enjoying their *kafe* in the morning, I've decided that the Greeks have figured out the secret to life! Any society that can manage to enjoy wine, cheese, good bread, and sunshine, all things that we are told may kill us (and then don't!), well, sign me up. They've done the impossible. Moderation. The gods were right. Not to mention the fact that my beloved latte was typically €1.50 in Greece, while now around $7 at home. Multiplying this by the number of lattes that I actually purchase in a calendar year does give one reason to pause.

I yearn to spend more time in Greece. Is part-time residence out of the question?! Having said that, I've identified two small, yet not insurmountable, downsides. First, there's the question of cost. Despite the decent (and surprisingly cheap) espressos, I'm acutely aware of the fact that I need to make more money. Travel seems to be rising in cost much like everything else, so this plan is going to require funding. The second downside is that, thanks to our rapidly warming globe, Greece, like many Mediterranean countries, seems to be consistently ablaze in the hotter months. Wildfires have fast become the norm through the summer. Now this aside, I'm thinking that I may just have to investigate further. It's going to take more than a few wildfires to deter me from this island paradise. If it's good enough for the gods, it's good enough for me. We have some of the finest beaches on the planet in Australia, but we also seem to have a considerable number of sharks in our waters, and from my modest knowledge of the Mediterranean, it seems to me that I have far less chance of being taken by a shark over there.

Alexander shares my feelings. Being a rather astute young man, Alex watched on with horror when we paid €50 for a five-minute taxicab ride somewhere on Naxos. He declared soon after, "Mummy, after I graduate high school, I'm moving to Greece to drive a car!" It took him all of two seconds in witnessing this transaction to realize that it would probably be better to be the person receiving the €50, rather than the one parting with it.

One curious and welcome surprise gift of our Greek sojourn was a temporary ceasing of my craving for sweets. Never in my life have I not wanted a gelato. However, after three weeks of walking, hiking, and sunset swimming in the

Aegean, I no longer craved sugar. This was a massive "aha!" moment. I realized that after three weeks of eating farm-fresh eggs, recently harvested fish, and marinated vegetables, and some local cheese and wine, I had successfully and inadvertently reset my tastebuds. For the first time in my life, I didn't want sugar. Fresh fruit was the exception—it still is. Once you've enjoyed a nectarine, perfectly sweet and dripping with juice at the height of summer, everything else pales in comparison.

I'm still surprised at how quickly my body responded to this new lifestyle. I'd spent decades trying desperately to achieve balance, some semblance of natural order within my body, and it turns out all I had to do was holiday in the Mediterranean, briefly embracing the local way of life. Who knew?!

What I know now is that when we eat refined sugar, we crave refined sugar, and when we eat Greek salad, we crave Greek salad. The body knows what it needs. If we're very still and listen, truly listen, our body will tell us what we need—and in no uncertain terms. There is an inherent wisdom in our cells, and to tap into that wisdom is truly life-changing. And on the flip side, if we eat crap, we feel like crap—and often crave more of it. I don't have to delve far back in time to recall that distinct sensation.

the way

*The secret to living well and longer is: eat half, walk
double, laugh triple, and love without measure.*

—Tibetan Proverb

Spain came next. The Camino de Santiago. Richard Branson's enthusiastic refrain has long inspired me to jump into adventures with wild enthusiasm. "Screw it, let's do it!" These were the words I heard as I booked three tickets to Madrid one rainy late autumn afternoon. My hunger for travel and adventure had only grown after our magical Greek odyssey, and never one to be worried about the practicalities of spending my savings, I decreed that we were going, come hell or high water. Anyway, life's far too short to waste time being practical. We had finally sold our oversized family home in Australia (years after the legal divorce) and as a result, I finally had the financial ability to travel again with the children. Hallelujah!

The Camino de Santiago is an ancient pilgrimage and series of walking routes, leading to the tomb of Saint James in the Santiago de Compostela, in northwest Spain. Becoming increasingly popular, this ancient pilgrim route is now extremely busy through the summer months; hence, I concluded that we would walk in March. Yes, we risked poor weather; however, we also avoided the crowds and competition for a bed at the end of a long day. Also bound by the constraints of the children's school schedules, we chose to complete the final and most popular section of the Camino, from Sarria to Santiago.

While wandering through the travel section of a quaint independent bookstore, I briefly glanced at a hiking book on the Camino de Santiago. This quickly snowballed into a concrete plan, sparking an idea that rapidly developed into a full-blown itinerary, my yearning for adventure insatiable.

"Yeah, I don't really think I want to get up every day and walk," was Cerulean's response. Three tickets it was.

"Are you serious?" Emily was wide-eyed.

Gasping in surprise, Alexander checked with me for confirmation before replying, "Yeah! I'd love to, Mummy!" Alex was on board in a heartbeat, quickly starting a mental packing list. He was an unusually organized fifteen-year-old, really. Then again, yes is Alexander's enthusiastic response to most things. Apples and trees . . .

"Okay. Let's do this!" I announced to my offspring, firm in my decree.

"You mean you walk it? Across the country?! Well, I might do one week, but that's it!" Emily was firm on this timeframe. Anything more seemed overwhelming, I suspect.

I grinned, unable to contain my enthusiasm.

"Seriously?" Incredulity from Emily. She was fascinated, and unaware that people would willingly choose to trek this distance voluntarily and call it a holiday. I think she was initially baffled by the whole concept.

The good news is that it turned out to be very easy to bribe a seventeen-year-old when the bribe was tempting enough. I'd always approved of the European attitude of introducing alcohol to children in a respectful, sensible manner. When has prohibition ever worked? Anywhere? With anything?!

So, there I was, well aware of this ace that I held, determined to convince the middle child that this was actually going to be fun (and when is anything an easy sell to a teenager?). I pressed on, explaining, "At the end of every day there are pilgrim meals that are served with red wine . . . for *everyone* . . ." I decided to take the direct approach when selling this multiday hike to my seventeen-year-old. Needless to say, when Emily realized that she would be able to enjoy red wine with her evening meal (and feel very grown up in the process), she eventually agreed to the journey. In fact, Emily made it clear to anyone who asked that this was the only reason that she agreed to the expedition. And who was I to argue? After all, people who tell us not to bribe kids don't have kids. I'm convinced that the authors of many a parenting book are secretly childless. Any parent worth their salt knows the value of a well-timed bribe.

Now, packing for the Camino, I made the classic beginner mistakes. You know the type . . . the ones that bloggers and YouTubers warn us of. Number one: don't overpack. I reasoned, of course, that my sturdy frame could more than handle a few extra pounds. What I didn't factor in was the reality of carrying these extra pounds on my now smaller frame, day in and day out. Turns out, shit gets heavy—and fast.

Having landed in Madrid, surviving the three connecting flights, and somewhat overcoming the jetlag, our collective excitement was beginning to build. After a pleasant train ride to Sarria and one more overnight to acclimatize, we hit the trail. Encountering a light rain the first morning left us all incredibly thankful for our wet weather outer layers.

The realization on day three that we had overpacked left me incredibly thankful for the Spanish postal service! So off we marched to find the nearest *oficina de correos*. Unfortunately, we were met with a lady whose grasp of the English language was just about as proficient as my Spanish (and she probably didn't have lead poisoning). In any event, Google Translate saved us more than once on this sojourn, I can tell you. We packed up a sturdy box of crap deemed superfluous, said a prayer, handed it over to the definitely-not-bilingual postal worker, and bid her good day. In Spanish!

You can imagine my joy when one month later my pink travel hairdryer arrived on my doorstep in Vancouver. I know, I know, a travel hairdryer on a hike. . . . This will likely seem ridiculous to many of you, however I'm not most people, and prior to this trip, the state of my hair was still a viable concern. By day two of the hike, I couldn't have cared less what my hair looked like. How quickly priorities can change! I failed in one regard, and that was in not remembering the following adage: When traveling, pack twice as much money and half as many clothes.

Is this ever bad advice? Not in my experience.

What was also curious was the speed with which food quickly became fuel for the trail. No longer something to obsess over, we were satiated in other ways. This journey also taught me that we all snack far more than we need to. Curiously, while walking, my body found its own natural equilibrium. I was at peace, the Spanish hillsides feeding my appetite for adventure that had been—prior to Greece—nothing more than an impractical fantasy. I was rarely hungry while walking during the daytime. Evening meals were enjoyed, my appetite kicking in at this point. I realized that I was allowing myself to eat intuitively, as we are meant to. I ate what my body needed to fuel the next day, no more or less. There were no crazy dieting rules or restrictions, simply pure enjoyment of movement in the daytime, good food in the evening, and restorative slumber through the night. I was in heaven. We all were.

As I write these words now, I ache to book our next hiking adventure through Europe! *Where and when?* I wonder. There's just something incredibly empowering about standing on a hillside, looking to the horizon, and then setting off by foot in that direction. The sense of achievement when arriving at the next village on the next hilltop was like nothing we had ever experienced before. We are meant to move— given legs for a reason! I pondered this realization. Humans aren't built to sit all day in an office chair, decade after decade. No wonder so many of us end up so very unhappy, overweight, depressed, anxious, and generally dissatisfied. Lives of quiet desperation indeed.

Now, an altogether different type of desperation hit my son and I in Spain, and early on in our travels too. You see, for some time now my children and I have consumed very little in the way of dairy products, switching to oat milk because we enjoyed the taste and had all found that less dairy generally equaled less blocked noses. A definite win given the dubious history with my sinuses. Mornings were something of a pilgrimage within a pilgrimage, in search of our morning *café con leche de avena* (coffee with oat milk). Perhaps not surprisingly, the deeper we trod into farming land, and the more cows we passed, the more we were greeted with, *"No. No avena!"* with disproval from the locals ranging from mild to severe. Now, not being one to actually survive without

coffee, and despising soy milk more than I do Tinder perverts, I made the switch back to cow's milk, as did my son.
And on the day that we also decided (unwisely, as it turns
out) to ingest Greek yogurt and cheese for lunch with our
baguette, plus gelato after dinner, we both discovered in no
uncertain terms that we are—without question—lactose
intolerant. Frequent bathroom trips are never fun, and when
the bathroom isn't your own, even less so—and no one needs
that in an *albergue* in a foreign country, let me tell you.

Turns out there's a limit to the local soft cheeses—or any
dairy, for that matter—that my son and I can enjoy without
taking those weird lactase tablets that assist in digestion.
Mind you, those tablets are vastly preferable to the colly-
wobbles, or what my children and I like to delicately call
fast poos, because when they hit, one can't get to the shared
albergue bathroom fast enough.

I'd long suspected that dairy was not my friend, and this
day was all the confirmation I needed. After all, Emily had also
consumed a huge amount of lactose that day and suffered no
ill effects. So there Alex and I were in Spain, having to seriously moderate our dairy consumption or suffer the rather
unpleasant consequences. Even the cows looked disappointed
as we trod past dairy after dairy. Mind you, being early spring,
the pungent aroma of manure was impossible to avoid, and
Emily's very audible protests may have contributed to their
morose demeanor. It's very possible that we were disturbing
the local herds with our colorful Australian vernacular.

The food on this holiday was outstanding, but it was
enjoyed in a balanced way, without the excesses, followed by
periods of restriction that I had known for so long. My body
had finally, after so many years, found the equilibrium that I
had been craving.

Our faces glowed with health and vitality. My son's acne, for months a source of anguish, naturally cleared up. My face became leaner, not gaunt. More healthy, alive. Sleeping deeply, we would awake to our new routine. Shower, pack, load everything onto our backs, and head out, following the yellow arrows and stopping at the first sign of *café con leche de avena* (on a good day!). There was magic in the simplicity, a calm and peace to our new rhythm. Never have I had such intense quality time with my children. Their iPhones also took a back seat to life, and with each slice of *tarta de Santiago*, I became more and more convinced that my children would never leave. Goodness knows I didn't want to go home either. The regional specialty of tarte made with ground almonds, eggs, and oranges fast become a staple on the trail, the calories needed when we were clocking thirty or forty thousand steps some days.

To maintain this state of equilibrium upon my return home, to the realities of day-to-day life, took conscious effort. Pause. Stop. Feel. Be Here Now. And then I asked myself, *What do I need right now? To satisfy physical hunger? Am I tired? Do I need a hug?* When I'm hungry, I eat. Called intuitive eating, it's surprising how quickly and naturally this happens when you spend time trekking across foreign lands. I didn't have to try in Spain. An ongoing challenge is finding this equilibrium at home when the typical stressors arise, when there is constant access to food and daily realities abound. It's constant work. Perhaps it always will be.

The Camino is often referred to as the Way. Not lost on me is the parallel with the spiritual teachings of Lao-tzu. In the *Tao te Ching*, he discusses the Tao (literally translated: the Way).

An absolute beginner when it comes to these teachings, I can only share what I have humbly (and recently) learned here. So please do be patient with me!

The Tao is all about balance, the middle way, where energy moves us forward and is not wasted, vacillating from one extreme to the other. Of course, I think of the extreme diets of my youth, the extreme exercise regimes. I was all out of balance, and about as far from Lao-tzu's Way as one could be. And I hear Apollo's call to moderation here, the parallels not lost on me. I discovered moderation in Greece and refined this in Spain while on the Way—discovering this quite by accident! The goal now is to maintain this balance, this moderation. And I'm getting better at it! Like anything, the more we practice something, the easier it becomes. Habit formation and maintenance continue to be integral for my physical and mental health (neuroplasticity at work . . . I could almost hear my synapses firing and wiring together while I slept!).

Many hike the Camino for deeply spiritual reasons. It is, after all, one of the three ancient pilgrimages (the other two being Rome and Jerusalem). Some now embark upon this pilgrimage for the love of hiking, others for varied health reasons and so forth. Curiously, the Pilgrim's Office in Santiago is keeping records of these reasons. Upon completing the hike, we were asked individually—before being given our certificates of completion—the reason for our walk. Turns out one of my kids answered, "I don't know."

Oh well.

Personally, I couldn't walk this trail without giving thought to the great beyond. Now, my father, being an atheist, was insistent that we be raised with no organized religion, despite my mother teaching Sunday School before her dramatic and rather rapid fall from grace. My grandmother was in her day a WASP: definitely white, definitely Anglo Saxon, and of course, Protestant. Anyway, as a result, I'm not christened.

"I want the girls to make up their own minds when they're old enough," declared my father, whenever the subject of religion arose (and let's be clear—that wasn't often). Fair enough, I could respect that logic. My grandmother was no doubt horrified. Not only was I the bastard grandchild, I was now also destined for a one-way ticket to hell. And then it hit me: Perhaps she didn't care? After all, her disdain for my existence was never hidden. Why would she care for the fate of my immortal soul?

Well, the joke's on her, because despite my lack of religious instruction or adherence to rules in general, I seem to be on very good terms with Saint James these days. And this is no small thing (I'm serious—I think he likes me). Not only one of the twelve apostles, Saint James the Greater was taken as the great protector of the Spanish soldiers when defeating the Moors, and is one of the patron saints of Spain to this day. Now, I'm not sure where he'd sit on the subject of my Javier liaison, given that my dear Javier is likely to have that hot Moorish blood running through his veins, but let's not dwell on that fact. After all, like the many before me, I walked the walk, offering up my ravaged feet at the site of his final resting place at the Compostela de Santiago. Of course, I do fear that my language alone may earn yours truly a speedy passage into the depths of hell, given that I tend to take the Lord's name in vain multiple times daily.

Now back to the subject of my being heard, and possibly even liked, by the great Saint James. A rather bold claim I realize. But here's why I dare make such a claim. Upon arrival at the Compostela, Emily, Alex, and I proceeded to pray. Let me elaborate. We walked in, tired, somewhat disheveled, but happy, and were met by the most spectacular cathedral that I have ever seen in my life. Words cannot begin to do this house of God justice, so I will refrain from trying.

"Oh wow. Oh. My. God." Looking up, Emily was in awe—and may also be destined to go down, not up, if blasphemy is any indicator of direction.

"*Shhhhhhhhhhh*," whispered Alex. "The sign says '*no talking*'!" said my ever-observant boy, still whispering. We nodded.

Ahead was an area for donations and an opportunity for weary pilgrims to light a candle and pray. Now my dear, fatigued children had walked a good 15 km that morning. They were hungry, weary, their feet blistered and aching, and all of us were in need of a hot shower. I'm reasonably confident that what they prayed for on that day was all three, the first being dinner. Spanish tapas.

My humble prayers ran just a little deeper.

"Mummy, can we go now?" Emmy whispered.

"Not yet. I'm still praying," I murmured with some force.

"*Shhhhhhhhhhh!*" said Alex.

Giving us both an excellent Paddington Bear hard stare, his eyes boring into our own, he admonished his sister.

"Emily, have some patience! Please!" I whispered in return, in a cranky, very ungodly way.

Back to my prayers. And in that moment, I gave thanks for the inordinate number of blessings in my life. And then I humbly asked for a great many things, the first regarding my troubled eldest child, Cerulean. Now what happened next can't possibly be a coincidence. You see, for several months throughout the pandemic, Cerulean struggled with an anxiety and depression so acute that they were often not able to get out of bed. They lost weight, they didn't shower, they didn't eat (why did that so rarely happen to me?!). I digress—it was horrific. As any parent who has navigated something similar will understand, to watch your child struggle so is the very definition of heartbreak. On that day in Spain, I prayed for Cerulean from the depths of my soul, and when we returned from Europe, I returned to a different child. Where there was darkness, there was now the beginnings of light. Of hope. And to this day they continue this upward trajectory, soon to begin university with a lust for life that I haven't seen in them for many, many years. And so yes, I do have faith in the great beyond, in a world after this one. And I don't doubt for a second that Saint James heard my prayers on that early spring day in Santiago in 2023.

the dogs

You have brains in your head. You have
feet in your shoes. You can steer yourself
any direction you choose.

—Doctor Seuss

"**A**rghhh!" Emily looked on, aghast. "Eww. Put the dogs away, Mummy, seriously. That is *so* disgusting!" This was my middle child's "compassionate" take on the state of my post-Camino feet.

"Thanks, Emily, but unfortunately the state of my dogs is quite out of my hands right now."

"Please don't ever say that again," Emily begged.

I think I did—and I shall henceforth refer to my feet as "dogs." If nothing else, it horrifies my children (and thereby amuses me). Apparently, no one in their forties is allowed to use the vernacular of today's youth. I seek to change that. Perhaps I can bridge the gap? And am I really that old?! After all, forty is the new thirty. And being that I'm only as old as the man I recently felt, I'm going with thirty-two. Enough said. But I digress. Again.

Anyway, my dear reader, upon our return to Vancouver, I also felt the need to pray for my toenails. Not quite as critical as my eldest child's metal health, but with summer coming, I had something of a problem. You see, I had the misfortune

172

to lose several toenails during our Spanish adventure, and my feet looked nothing short of revolting that spring. And it turns out that one's toenails take an inordinate amount of time to regrow. Who knew? My first step was ridding myself of the ill-fitting shoes. Then it was off to the local outdoor store.

Tackling the Vancouver traffic, which is a feat in itself, I found myself in one of my happy places. Surrounded by a veritable treasure trove of brightly colored and very practical goodies for my outdoor sojourns, I surveyed the store and smiled. Something about an outdoor store always inspires my next adventure—and a need for more hiking socks. One never can have too many pairs. Mine always seem to go missing, to be found on the feet of my offspring . . . hence the need to constantly replenish.

"The general rule of thumb is an extra thumb's width at the front of the hiking boot!" espoused the young salesman, bouncing with energy as if about to complete a Camino of his own. Excellent. This would have been helpful knowledge prior to our multiday trek. *But oh well, better late than never,* I reasoned. Now the only family member to return from the hike with all ten toenails was my youngest, who hiked in Italian boots. My mind was made up. It was Italian hiking boots or none.

This led me to the next problem with my impending purchase. Statistically, Australians have among the widest feet on the planet (yes, somebody has evidently researched this). My theory is that we are all barefoot for so many days of our childhood down there—at least I was—that our feet naturally widen without the arch support of sensible shoes. It's all rather unfortunate, because the cute, girly pale-blue hiking boots did not come in my size. Ditto the pink. Ugh.

"I'm very sorry. We don't seem to stock that size."

I see. Well, given that I wasn't about to board a flight to Italy to purchase the hiking boots of my dreams, a decision had to be made.

"Some women find that a men's boot fits them better, particularly if their foot is a little wider."

Terrific. I'd worked out like a fiend to have the petite ass of my dreams, and still I'm destined to have huge man-like feet. Well, I suppose it could be worse. Imagine if I'd been born into one of those Asian cultures, where they bind your feet to ensure they remain tiny. I would have been seriously fucked.

So anyway, I left the store on that sunny spring day having lost and gained. I was many hundreds of dollars poorer, but I gained the most comfortable pair of hiking boots that I've ever worn. And I'm pleased to report that they're in a lovely Sensible Susan shade of brown. Again, there is a God.

The Camino also gave my children the gift of movement. We may have lost a few toenails, but what we gained was so much more. Alex and Emily now both see distance differently—everything is relative, after all. A 10-km walk is nothing to them now, and they voluntarily choose to walk when the weather is good. I need to stress at this point that Emily is the same girl who would once complain of boredom after 200 m on a local hiking trail (and complain at length about how walking sucked, like only a teenager can). Well, not anymore! I have gifted my children with the priceless joy of movement, of travel and exploration of foreign lands. The world is broad and wide, and my (mostly grown) children are now eager to explore more of it. For this I will be forever grateful.

It's interesting that now distance is relative—the kids having gained a whole new perspective when it comes to the reality of 1, 5, or 10 km—I can move forward, planning future expeditions, safe in the knowledge that they are more than capable. After all, they've done 30 km in a day (at a push) with a huge pack on their backs through early spring rain, wind, and mud. We will continue to adventure! I firmly believe that it is my duty as a mother to help my children build resilience. The world isn't always easy to navigate, and the sooner they learn this, the better. Quite frankly, if hiking with a huge pack through rain and wind with lactose-induced diarrhea doesn't build resilience, then I don't know what does.

shame

*You will never do anything in this world
without courage. It is the greatest quality
of the mind next to honor.*

—Aristotle

When I left my husband, I had this innate feeling, perhaps without conscious realization, that I was trusting in something bigger. The universe, the gods, faith in something. Or was it faith in my capacity and abilities as a woman to get shit done? Quite possibly, all of the above. After all, I had no money, no separate bank account in my own name, no car in my own name, and no career at the time, save the title of Career Housewife, which earned precious little respect in the wider world.

"What do Mummy and Daddy do?" my Emily was asked once as a small child by an inquisitive kindergarten teacher.

"Daddy goes to the mine and Mummy does nothing!" Spoken with such earnest innocence.

Is this view changing? Yes, however slowly. There's still huge stigma associated with choosing full-time motherhood. Homemaker. Domestic engineer. Housewife. Kept woman. Loaded titles, and with them an assumption of privilege. And please don't get me wrong, I am very aware of the financial privilege required to have the luxury of choosing to remain at home and out of the paid workforce while one's children are young. I have nothing but respect for the phenomenal women who juggle motherhood with paid work outside of the home. I honestly don't know how people do it and remain sane. Lord knows, I struggled at times to wash my hair. Dressing for and driving to an office for eight hours a day seemed just about as realistic as manning a shuttle to the moon. And what woman with small children has the time to worry about her hair? Or the energy?!

Recently I showed my wild Australian teens an old photo. It was me, at possibly my biggest. We were on the precipice of another move, and the decades-old photo albums were unearthed during the packing process. Everyone was happy. We were moving to a tenth-floor apartment. Finally, a view! The irony of my former bunker-basement refuge was not lost on me, the move up in elevation mirroring the upward trajectory in other areas of my life.

"Oh my God. Is that you?!" was the initial response of Emily upon seeing an old photo. She audibly gasped. "No way. It's not. That can't be you!"

"That doesn't even look like you!" said Alex. Eyes wide, it was impossible for my children to contain their shock. "No way!"

No, it didn't look like me. But it was. And I've conveniently left these pictures securely stowed away, hidden in a low-profile storage tub under my bed, far away from the curious eyes of my lovers. As I look at these, I notice with curiosity how every photo immediately brings to mind a number: my weight at that point in my life. Always the number. And always associated with my worth, the number determining whether this would be a good day or bad, the bathroom scales holding far too much power for far too long.

So what was my biggest fear with these photos? Rejection, of course. That I wouldn't be loved. That my current boyfriend would no longer find me attractive. Desirable. Beautiful. How incredibly sad. I recognize as I write these words that for the longest time, I've held deep shame around the fact that I allowed myself to gain so much weight. It is only now with compassion that I look back and see an insecure young girl. A girl with parents who were also struggling to get through the day. A girl who ached to be loved, accepted, and cherished unconditionally.

And good news—now she is. By herself.

When you're a kid you don't realize that you're also watching your parents grow up.

Cerulean did, astutely commenting once, "Mummy, I think you've really matured a lot in the last few years. You're much wiser now!"

"Thank you, C. B. What a beautiful thing to say. And you know, I think I have too."

Cerulean was right. Completing postgraduate studies in psychology was instrumental in my continued growth and maturity. There's an inner calm now, whereas decades prior there was anxiety, restlessness, and a lack of self-confidence.

A life lived in fear is a life half-lived, and I just knew that I was not destined to live half a life. Shame and fear. Fear and shame. Intertwined when I think about my past physical body. Sure, my old Aussie friends and dearest Canadian girlfriends knew that there used to be more of me to love (far more), but in my present life, I have deliberately excluded this piece of information from my narrative—until now.

I help my clients overcome fear and resistance on a daily basis. It occurred to me that in writing this memoir, I was facing my greatest fear, and to do anything less would be inauthentic. How could I possibly counsel people facing their fears if I was unwilling to face mine?

sorry

No one can make you feel inferior
without your consent.

—Eleanor Roosevelt

Fat people apologize. A lot. I swear to God, I think I spent a good two decades apologizing. "Sorry. Sorry. I'm so sorry." And I was sorry—for everything. When a fat person apologizes, what they are really saying is, "I'm sorry for being here, for existing, for taking up space. For being me."

Sorry for my thighs.

Sorry for my childhood.

For my father.

For everything.

A blanket apology. Society has told us that we aren't good enough, so we try and make amends, starting with one continual apology.

"Jane, you say sorry a lot. I wonder, have you noticed that?"

"Jane, stop apologizing!"

"Jane, do you know that you apologize a lot? All the time, in fact?"

Well yes, I did realize that. My friends pointed this fact out on a regular basis. But it didn't stop the regretful acknowledgment of my failure to be thin. I'm sorry.

How was it that my self-worth could be tied so intimately to a single number: the digits on my bathroom scale? Numbers with the ability to bring joy or despair on any given day. Elation or frustration. When did I give away this power? When did a number begin to define my inherent worth? My value? My self-esteem? Decades ago, it turns out, and no longer will I allow this. While the bathroom scale is still a tool I utilize, ultimately my jeans will tell me if I've gained or lost a few pounds. I don't need an overpriced body-fat-composition monitor to tell me if they will or won't do up comfortably. It's really very simple when you think about it. Are my pants too tight? Yes/No. Do I want to change this? Yes/No.

Body dysmorphia can be defined as a disorder characterized by intrusive and negative thoughts relating to the appearance of one's body that are not consistent with the perceptions of other people. A great many people who have lost considerable amounts of weight then find themselves with new and surprising challenges. This first one is the excess skin. Not pretty. The second one is dysmorphia. I struggled with both, and the dysmorphia can still creep in some days if I'm not careful. This speaks to the power of the mind. I used to struggle to see that the woman staring back at me in the bathroom mirror was me. The challenge now is not to obsess—something we all know that I'm rather prone to do (it's one of my former specialties). Whether it was a boy or the size of my thighs, I was in a league of my own. Seriously, if there's a university out there somewhere handing out honorary doctorates for talents in obsessive thoughts, I should really get in touch with them. I was the poster child. It would have been impressive if it wasn't so destructive.

Clothes shopping felt somewhat surreal for the first few years after my weight loss. I'd automatically grab a medium or a large from the clothes rack, and the salesperson would have to correct me.

"Oh no, that's way too big on you. Here, try this . . ."

Handing me a small, I was constantly baffled. It looked so small! Was she sure?!

"Are you sure?!" I'd exclaim, not able to hide my surprise.

"Yes!" The salesgirl's surprise was also evident.

"Most people choose one size too small; you're choosing too large!" the lady exclaimed, perplexed. Only I knew why. Body dysmorphia is very real, and I was living with it daily in those early years.

My kids, in their brutal honesty, remain helpful when I'm in doubt. After returning home with one of those ruffled, floral maxi dresses (that I love), Alexander, God bless him, said the most helpful thing. Looking at me a little anxiously, his eyes and mouth were an expression of uncertainty. With a maturity beyond his years, he spoke the truth where the salesgirl did not.

"Ahh . . . I think it makes you look bigger than you are, Mummy."

"Thank you for your honesty, Alex," I replied.

The dress was returned for a full refund the following morning. After all, when isn't honesty preferable to the alternative? Despite my body acceptance at this point in my life, I had no desire to look larger than I was. Does anyone?! And is it wrong to feel this way?!

So many questions.

Very recently, I'd started wearing an oversized white hoodie (courtesy of my fickle children who wore it for five minutes, discarded it, and immediately informed me that I looked like a rap star's girlfriend when I decided to save it from the donation pile). Quite frankly, it's enormous. But here's the thing—it's *so* comfortable! And it occurred to me that it doesn't matter what I look like to the outside world, if I look large or small. Who the hell cares? I cared for so long, obsessed. No more would I obsess over my external form, and I swear to God, this is one of the most empowering epiphanies that I've ever had.

Time is healing. Finally at peace, comfortable in my body after decades at war. And how I enjoy shopping for new clothes now—a little too much, if I'm being honest. I can finally buy and wear exactly what I wish, no longer relegated to the far corner of the store where the plus sizes reside in the shadows, as if also apologizing for their presence.

Yes, things are changing, slowly. I still recall my shock the first time I passed a Victoria's Secret and saw a plus model in the window. Wow. We really have evolved since the waif-crazed '90s. And how wonderful and empowering for women everywhere. I'm filled with relief when I think of my own children, praying that they never endure the pain of disordered eating. To see bodies of all shapes and sizes in storefronts and magazines is a wonderful step in the right direction. Never do I want my children to feel what I felt. That they aren't enough. That they need to stop eating. That they need to throw up after a large meal in order to be loved. To be worthy. To be enough.

Because they are enough. We all are, by virtue of being human.

We are all enough.

acceptance

You are the sky. Everything else is just the weather.

—Pema Chödrön

The mountains of Wyoming, wild and spectacular, loomed before me as I stretched, soaking up the sunshine deep into my bones. Standing by the oversized glass windows, I looked out, drinking in the solidity and calm. The appropriately named Heart Mountain was to my right.

Time for work! As I sat at my laptop, typing and reflecting upon my life thus far, I was taking stock.

"Did you know that Hemmingway wrote some of his best work in Wyoming?" asked Dr. A.

"I'm not surprised," I replied. After all, the landscape was nothing short of inspirational. I was in good company. If Wyoming assisted the late, brilliant Ernest Hemmingway to pen some of America's greatest literary works, I figured my humble memoir could also benefit from the spectacular natural beauty that surrounded me. Mind you, Hemmingway was reported to have written until noon, at which point he'd start drinking the afternoon away. Not wishing to develop this particular affliction, I abstained, save the odd glass of red with dinner.

The visits to my paramour had become sabbaticals. I'd read and write. We'd cook, make love, play indoors and out as we explored the beautiful and empty desert biking trails. It was paradise, my escape from an increasingly unpleasant urban world that I called home. The vastness, the friendly townsfolk, and the lack of traffic reminded me of my youth and the wild big-sky country that I left behind so many years before.

Australia.

How far I'd come. I was acutely aware that many of my childhood friends never left that dusty town, choosing an early marriage to a local boy and babies, their worlds kept small and safe. While I also elected to marry early and dive into motherhood, that was never going to be enough, always knowing that my path would somehow be so much more, that I would demand more of life. And that I'd get the hell out of Broken Hill.

Without change, we stagnate. Change is truly the only constant in life, yet the one thing humans inherently resist. I see it in my practice every day. People unable to accept the inevitability of change. Unwilling to accept that most things in life are absolutely and completely out of our control. They fight against it, resisting. Anxiety and depression often follow. Eckhart Tolle tells us in *The Power of Now* that all pain stems from resistance to what is. How right he is. Acceptance is the only path—it was for me. I changed what I could and accepted the remainder. The alternative? Pain. Frustration. Energy wasted as we try in vain to fight against reality, living in the past or the future where we know anxiety and depression to live.

Paradoxically, when I was able to truly accept my reality, I was then able to change. Acceptance was the path to my freedom. Joy and a calm mind are the spoils, at peace in the present moment. And sure, I'm human and imperfect. We all are. Some days it's harder to remain grounded in the present, and that's okay. Through embracing self-compassion, I'm able to care for myself with a gentleness that I didn't know possible a few years ago. I do wonder, *How different would my life have been, had I learned these tools, these lessons at a younger age? If my insecure teenaged self had had access to this knowledge?*

Embodiment. Interoceptive awareness. Perhaps the most powerful tool of all for the recovering emotional eater. Allow me to pause here and expand upon this for a moment. Essentially, interoceptive awareness is the perception of sensations from within the body. To feel your heartbeat, the fullness in your stomach, the sensation of a breath, the in and out of the lungs. Through this practice we facilitate a reconnection of mind and body. My eating disorder had little if nothing to do with true physical hunger and everything to do with a disconnection from my physical body. I was essentially dissociated from internal sensations of fullness as I attempted to escape from my life, briefly avoiding reality and its accompanying responsibilities.

The healing began with yoga, before I had any awareness of the path I had begun to tread. This was no small piece of the puzzle, as yoga allowed a reconnection of my mind with my body. A journey of healing and recovery. One person actually asked me if I'd had gastric band surgery.

"How *did* you lose the weight? And how do you keep it off?" one nurse enquired, unable to hide her surprise at my tale, the before and after statistics, the morning of my tummy tuck as she took my blood pressure.

I thought about my answer, pausing. *How did I do it?* "Persistence. Determination. And key was addressing the

hungers, none of which were physical. Plus, a *lot* of exercise."
(Still nonnegotiable to keep from regaining.)

If this sounds simplistic, it is and it isn't. Healthy food, exercise, moderation, and a thorough rejection of the insanity that is modern-day diet culture. Are some days still a challenge? Of course. But this is how I did it. The first step was figuring out just why I was emotionally eating. I had to figure out what I was hungry for, because it sure as hell wasn't food.

When interviewed after her very public weight loss, Adele reported that perhaps she was meant to be an athlete, addressing her newfound love of exercise. I could relate. After two decades of largely being inactive, my physical body also awoke. As a child I had enjoyed team sports, and then the brutal teenage years hit. Many girls ceased participation in organized sports, only the elite continuing on at higher levels of competition. Certainly, in my youth, mediocrity wasn't encouraged. If you weren't the best, you tended to bow out.

Combining this newfound lack of physical activity with my growing eating disorder, well, the results were disastrous for my waistline. I remember the ridiculous wholemeal bread diet. I was around fourteen years old when I embarked upon this first diet with my mother. It was very simple really. Every second day, we were to eat nothing but whole wheat bread. Madness. I also remember the egg and apple diet that my mother spoke of, circa 1976. Not sure what that would have achieved other than possibly some very unfortunate Amanda Wilson-style farts. But of course, I tried them all. And they worked until they didn't. Because diets don't work. The deep-seated emotional causes of my comfort eating were never addressed, and as a result any form of restriction was doomed to fail. And fail it did.

"Laura, when are you going to lose some weight like your sister?!" my father asked once in exasperation.

Poor Laura. My sister had similar but different challenges. Emotional eating for sure, but combined with several anti-seizure drugs that likely wreaked havoc with her growing body.

Dad, in a rare moment of attentiveness in my late teens, had noticed that for once, one of my dieting efforts had finally achieved some measure of success: protein drinks and walking. The restriction worked, briefly, combined with my ironclad willpower to finally shed some weight. I longed to shop for the cute teenaged clothes of my friends. I wore so many navy fleece tracksuits back in those days, my friends christened me Navy Spice of the Spice Girls. Really, I looked like Frumpy Spice, and I felt very much like this. I was far from a Spice Girl. Ironically, at least two Spice Girls have spoken about their eating disorders at the height of their fame. I'm yet to find one person surprised by this revelation. How could we be? They had no choice but to starve or binge and purge to maintain a physique their management would have demanded back then. Sex sells. Fat doesn't.

Without realizing it at the time, this was my first experience with positive habit formation. I'd purchased a book on the benefits of walking and concluded that I'd walk my way to health. It was 1997, and while not extremely overweight, I was certainly carrying more weight than was healthy for my sturdy frame. Naturally the movement was effective. I'd wanted to purchase a treadmill initially, reasoning that I could walk under the air-conditioning and in the privacy of my own home. One small but real problem was my lack of funds.

My father, pointing to the front door, put it best. "You see that path leading to the front gate, Jane?" he asked.

"Yes," I replied.

"Right then. You walk down there, out the front gate, turn left, and keep going. There's your treadmill!" Laughing at his own joke, I feigned annoyance. Secretly I was amused, as he was correct.

So, I took his advice (possibly for the first time) and didn't look back. To this day I prefer to walk outdoors when at all possible.

My daily constitutional fast became a happy habit. My dog, Clive, and I would set out in the direction of the golf club, a pleasant 6-km return trip. Nothing crazy, just consistent movement. My enthusiastic Corgi-cross was always wildly excited upon departure, and consistently tired upon the return journey. His little legs would tire on the last home stretch, which was slightly uphill. My sturdy legs could have continued—they do to this day, I suppose.

As for my father, I made peace with him long ago. The Buddha was right: Forgiveness is the only way. Acceptance. Because to accept something isn't necessarily to like it. We don't have to like what we accept; however, to accept is to make peace with *what is*, what cannot be changed, and what has long passed. And there's infinite power in acceptance. Forgiveness. And love.

Always love.

hummus

Everything in excess is opposed to nature.

—Hippocrates

Not too long after manifesting the lovely Dr. A, I had the misfortune of experiencing a moment in time reminiscent of the diet pills discomfort of my youth. Suffice to say, the timing couldn't have been worse. There we were, my new paramour and I, out for the afternoon on a mountain bike ride. And yes, much like Broken Hill, the hills of Wyoming are rather remote, isolated, and spectacular in their rugged beauty. And that's all well and good, provided that you are in good health. Well, it seems on that fateful day I would have done well to take my mother's advice many years ago regarding first dates.

Setting a good pace on our carbon bikes (acutely aware that my newly purchased bike cost considerably more than my first car), I was feeling both invigorated and energetic when disaster struck. I was suddenly overcome with a rather uncomfortable pain in my abdomen. I pushed on, dismissing it, until it intensified.

"Ahh, Dr. A, I'm not feeling so well. I have this pain. It's a tummy ache . . ."

Now, I'm sure at this point he may have been wondering, *Does she just not want to ride today?* Answer: Yes, I did, having truly fallen in love with this new activity.

"I'm okay, I'll keep going!" I hollered, channeling my inner Rowlf the Muppet in order to be heard, as he was up ahead now.

I pressed on. The pains intensified, and I was forced to stop. Now I would like to mention here that after thrice giving birth, I know what pain is, and my tolerance is high. And this was getting worse. Dr. A started to look concerned. He knew I wasn't one to quit. By now I was immobile and doubled over in pain.

"Do you want to stay here, and I'll go get the truck?" At this point we were several miles out of town, it was isolated, and I was well aware that a few days ago a grizzly bear was shot and killed close to our location. So that was a hard no.

"I'll be okay," I winced, forcing a smile.

Mercifully, the remaining trail was downhill, and very gingerly I climbed onto Puff my Magic Mountain Bike (aptly named for its purple and silver color and the magic I feel when rolling over boulders) and slowly attempted to roll back to town. Dr. A was asking the questions that only a doctor knows to ask. His fear was appendicitis, I later discovered.

"Where is the pain exactly? How sharp? Press here . . ." etc. The pain was intense.

He knew the general surgeon on duty that day in his small town, and so I reasoned that I'd die another day, unlike the grizzly.

We made it home. I stumbled to the bed and collapsed in pain. At this point I wasn't saying much. The pain was all consuming. Knowing me to be something of a talker, Dr. A was likely thinking, *This can't be good.* . . . I lay down, like a cat that retreats when ill, silent and immobile. Quiet isn't exactly my default setting.

Dr. A began to palpate my stomach, doing doctor things that only a doctor really understands.

Hmm.

He continued to investigate my newly flat (and bloody sore!) abdomen. Time passed. Evidently there was a hollow sound, and I heard him mutter about the descending colon. I'd like to mention that the day before, I did eat an inordinate amount of hummus and raw vegetables. I'm still not sure why.

"Well, I think you probably just need to fart," he concludes.

Oh. My. God.

Mortified, I lay there. Evidently my digestive system was not thrilled at the copious quantity of raw vegetables and hummus I downed the day prior. "Wind" to us Aussies, or the more delicately termed "pop-offs" to my grandmother.

I could have died, and not from the wind. Trapped gas the probable diagnosis.

Now there's a time in every relationship where this would be something to laugh about with ease and comfort. We weren't there yet—I certainly wasn't! In this early stage of our courtship, I was still wearing makeup. Good Lord. Not to mention blow-drying my hair. For the love of God! I sure as hell wasn't ready to discuss farts. And the lesson here? Your mother is usually right.

"Don't eat hummus before a first date, Jane!" she'd cautioned me years back.

I'd like to add to this wisdom. Just don't eat hummus.

Ever.

gratitude

Wear gratitude like a cloak and it will feed every corner of your life.

—Rumi

Sitting in my favorite cozy coffee shop writing this book, I'm aware that I've gained a couple of pounds. After a decade of maintaining this new healthy weight, I try and reconcile this gain through a lens of self-compassion. Do the two pounds I see on my thighs make me any less worthy? Less lovable? No, fuck it, they do not. And to hell with anyone who thinks otherwise. My weight does tend to bounce up and down a few pounds with the seasons, dependent largely on how much lactose-free cheese and wine I enjoy in any given month. And that's okay. Mine are not the wild fluctuations of the stock exchange. Frankly, it could be a whole lot worse.

The scientific community never can seem to agree on much. Having said that, the consensus seems to be that the majority of people who have once been overweight or obese and lose the weight usually gain most, if not all, of it back. Many within twelve months, and almost all within five years. These sobering statistics paint a rather bleak picture. Many even gain a little extra, finding themselves at a higher weight than their initial number. It's all rather depressing really. The good news is that a small percentage do keep the weight off long-term, and I count myself lucky to be among their numbers. But I know it's not luck. It's hard bloody work! My hope, in writing this book, is that anyone for whom this will relate to can walk away with hope in knowing that if I can lose the weight and keep it off for a decade, anyone can. I want to share what I've learned: Weight loss is possible without extreme gastric band surgery, stomach stapling, Ozempic, diet pills, or one thousand other drastic external and internal interventions. And I know that this is possible—because I did it.

I do wish to humbly share a few words of wisdom, the knowledge that I have acquired this past decade. First, we cannot change what we don't accept. A paradox, yes, however when we truly love and accept ourselves as we are, then we are able to change. Grow. Heal. Transform. Thrive. I had to begin by owning my body. My weight. All of it.

Second, be gentle with yourself, because Lord knows, the world won't be. It is imperative that you be your own best friend. Starting now. And this is how: You begin by asking yourself, "What do I want right now? At this very moment in time? What do I need right now?" I ask myself this a lot. And the answer varies. Sometimes it's a hot bath. Sometimes I want to go to bed. Sometimes I want to escape to the mountains to hike. Sometimes it's nourishing food. And now here's the second instruction: Do it. Have it. Deprivation doesn't work. Ever.

And third—here's the thing. We are all going to die. Probably not tomorrow, but at some point, it's inevitable— the one thing we are all guaranteed. Who was it who said that no one gets out of this alive? Indeed.

Now when we realize and truly accept this reality, we can start living. Really living. The kind of "fuck it" living that makes you realize that it doesn't matter what your mother-in-law said that was hurtful. What the waiter said when he told you that you'd ordered the biggest main on the menu (so rude). Your thighs that aren't Instagram smooth. Fuck it all. And who the bloody hell cares anyway?! My body has birthed three phenomenal children. I'm not a nubile eighteen-year-old. I'm forty-five and counting. How in the name of God can anyone expect me to have the smooth, delightful thighs of a teenage girl? And guess what? I stopped worrying, stopped obsessing. Fuck it. My legs are strong, they work, they carry me up a mountain when I hike. And for that I am grateful.

Gratitude. It's a gamechanger. Because the minute that we are grateful for what we have, we lose focus of all the wants. They fall away. Everything that we don't have and invariably think we need. For many this includes the unrealistic, empty desire for our youth. The perfect skin, wrinkle free, toned thighs, hair thick and lustrous. Would having this again bring happiness? No.

Sure, I'd love physical perfection for five minutes, but it's an illusion. And if we're dissatisfied internally, it counts for naught.

bananas

Let food be thy medicine and medicine be thy food.

—Hippocrates

t's a very curious thing, the way that people everywhere feel that they have the right to comment on another person's body. This has been a common theme throughout my life. The thing is, I'll always be sturdy, and at the age of forty-five, I've finally made peace with this fact. And I now truly love my body. Hell, I'm just so grateful that it's stuck by me, after everything I've put it through.

And I love food. I still love food. I've *always* loved food. I'm a foodie! (And, mercifully, a failed anorexic.) The difference now, at this point in my life, is that I also respect food. I respect my body. I want to also set the right example for my children while teaching them to enjoy food—the flavors, the textures, the different cuisines. I truly believe that food is one of life's joys and must be respected. I aim to remind myself of this daily. My goal now is balance and moderation in all things. Apollo was right. Moderation. And when I practice this, I find I can enjoy bread, wine, and cheese. Just not in unhealthy excess.

Grandmother had some odd views, like many of her generation. (And this generation! Who am I kidding?!) "Bananas will make you fat, Jane! And so will whole grain bread!" Really? Hmm. I'm pretty sure that the world's obesity epidemic hasn't been brought on by excess banana consumption. In fact, I'm quite certain of that. I've managed to maintain my considerable weight loss for a decade now, and I have done so while eating both bananas and grain bread, on an almost daily basis. I do concede that too much bread isn't ideal; however, I prefer Apollo's views on moderation to include bread, in all of its heavenly, fresh-out-of-the-oven glory.

Let me expand on this controversial, much-loved, and shunned staple for a moment. I am convinced that mass-produced supermarket bread is absolute crap. I'd rather go without. What I do enjoy in moderation is an organic, locally milled, unleavened bread from my nearby bakery. Their sourdough is food for the gods—and for my very appreciative children. And if there's a world that exists without sourdough, well, I have no desire to live in it.

Here's another relevant fact—food always tastes better when we're hungry. So let yourself feel hungry! Get hungry. Be hungry. It's okay. You won't die, and I guarantee that when you sit down for a meal, it's going to taste just that much better because you *are* hungry.

"Hunger is the best sauce!" a wise eighteen-year-old once told me. And it's true. To eat when we're not hungry is downright uncomfortable. And if you weren't hungry to begin with, how on Earth will you know when you're full? We've all been there. I recall in my maternity days feeling overfull, my pants held together with a safety pin and a prayer. And I sure as hell recall feeling uncomfortable.

"*Uuugghhhhh.* Let me guess. A warm salad?" Emily was less than excited at the evening's offering.

"Correct!" Smiling at Emily, I confirmed her suspicions. Yes, in 2023, all manner of warm salads were on heavy rotation in our humble household.

"*Whyyyyyyyyy?*" Emily was prone to extending one word into several, as you may have noticed.

"Emily, you've seen the before pictures. You've all seen the photos. If we ate creamy pasta dishes every night, my ass would be the size of England." I refuse to mince words.

Alex attempted to hide a giggle. He failed, and I suspect my formerly large derriere would be amusing to any fifteen-year-old boy. I realize that this speaks to a larger problem in society, but I also realize that Alex has inherited my wicked, dark sense of humor. And I can laugh about it now; I'm allowed to—it was my body, after all, and the children have no memory of me at a larger size, too young to recall my too tight pants.

I refuse to sugarcoat weight loss for my children (no pun intended). While appreciating that mine is a balancing act, between modeling healthy habits and ensuring I don't promote eating disorders in my offspring, I remain honest with them. The sky is blue, and if we eat too much unhealthy food and don't exercise enough, our pants won't fit. This remains a fact, and I believe that sharing this knowledge with my children is imperative. And as a result, I cook from scratch most evenings, with fresh whole foods that are largely plant-based. I try to keep the sugar down in recipes. And despite Emily's protests, I think she secretly likes my warm quinoa, spinach, and roasted beet salad.

Now much like processed white supermarket bread and refined sugar, I'd always thought astrology to be a complete and utter load of crap. Until I didn't. After all, it's not scientific! This was certainly the view in my twenties. Garbage. And then I started reading. And observing. Now I'm a Scorpio and a water sign, and many of my nearest and dearest friends are also earth and water signs. Coincidence? Perhaps. Or not. The brilliant Carl Jung was a believer, and who am I to argue with one of the fathers of modern psychology? Now I'm aware that some of you reading this will be in the load-of-crap camp, some ambivalent, and some of you will know not only where Mercury is right now, you will also know how the current moon may be affecting you and what is and isn't in retrograde. Either way, please humor me and allow this indulgence. I recently learned that a lesser-known symbol of Scorpio is the phoenix, in addition to the scorpion. And I love it. The perfect metaphor for my life. After all, didn't I voluntarily burn to ashes and rise, phoenix-like, from the smoke? I'd like to think yes. At least I'm humbly attempting this resurrection.

Death and rebirth. Transformation. More mature, wiser. No longer the insecure girl who vomited in her best friend's front hedge after seeing her in-laws, due to the anxiety that the visit triggered. That girl has transformed into the woman that she is today. And let me assure you, not even an earthquake can shake me too much at this point (literal shaking aside). I've just handled a lot. Once you've dealt with police cars at your rental basement suite not once, but twice, investigating possible child abuse, well, most else does seem to pale in comparison.

"You don't seem like a Scorpio." I've heard this many times.

Ahh, well, perhaps I keep that side of myself hidden from view. After all, Scorpios are known for secrecy. Depth, a dark intensity. It's been hidden for good reason. Until now I suppose.

Now Brian is a Gemini. We were the worst match in the zodiac. I do respect the fact that he's in the load-of-crap camp when it comes to astrology, as was I when we met; hence I didn't really give it a second thought. Was this the reason our marriage failed? No, of course not. Were we, in some ways, on two separate planets? Yes. Vows made too young, I had to break them. And when I broke them, I became whole.

grounded

Wherever there is a human being,
there is an opportunity for kindness.

—Seneca

To be grounded within oneself is essential for lasting change, and to truly find peace within our bodies is nothing short of life-changing. As I write these words at 3:00 a.m., my dearest Dr. A sleeps soundly beside me, and I reflect upon this monumental (and rather recent) shift. When did it happen? This peace I speak of, this calm? How, after a lifetime of fighting with my body, the recent years of maintenance, and occasional moments of regression? Sure, a bad day now might look like a bowl of sugar-laden granola, tummy ache–inducing ice cream, and toast with apricot jam (still a favorite) eaten when not hungry (of course). At least not hungry for food. Fortunately, these days are now rare—a once-a-year-holy-shit-meltdown day. And let's not forget that pleasure of all pleasures—the twice-baked almond croissant. Seriously, whoever invented this culinary delight deserves some type of award. Please, let's find this visionary so that they may be celebrated for their genius. Is there anything yummier?!

Calm. How *did* I achieve it at the age of forty-five, and I mean true calm within myself? The type of secure, solid, anchored-at-my-core calm that I have never before felt? This was my 3:00 a.m. question. And then how to share this with my clients so that they may also experience this groundedness that I now know to be imperative to finding peace within our bodies, to remain calm within the storms that life will inevitably throw at us.

Only once in my life have I been white water rafting. This excellent adventure took place in the Rocky Mountains of British Columbia, and it occurred to me soon afterward that this experience is much like life itself. There were periods of calm as we floated along, the sunshine restorative on our faces. A slight breeze, the early warmth promising a hot day ahead. And then the bend in the river, the rapids, danger. Unpredictable, exhilarating, requiring focus to navigate as we followed the instructions of our Australian guide (of course he was Australian! Where there is adventure to be had, we do tend to be found as a people). And at this point all you can do is hold on and trust that there are calm waters up ahead. Isn't life much the same?

To feel grounded within the madness and magnificence of it all—that's the game changer. And how do we do this? By truly accepting that most things in life are entirely and completely out of our control and then taking responsibility and ownership of the things that we can control. Think about it. When I wake tomorrow morning, or see the sunrise if I happen to be sitting here typing, how much is within my control? Precious little, that's how much. Can I control the weather? The irate driver who endangers us all with their reckless speeding? Can I control the lady at the grocery store who may or may not be having the worst day of her life? Can I control the phone call that will inevitably come one day, telling me that Laura is in the hospital again, suffering with delusions? No, I can't. But I can sure as hell control my response. My actions. And in doing so, my state of mind.

I control my response. Because here's the thing: When we are grounded at our core, and I mean truly grounded, the road-rage driver doesn't send us flying into our own indignant rage. Like the magic words as a child (still please and thank you!), the magic isn't really magic at all. It's acceptance, compassion, gratitude, and kindness. Acceptance of the fact that most of these external factors in our world are completely and entirely out of our control. Compassion for the challenges of the cranky lady at the supermarket who's struggling in her own world . . . at least today in aisle four.

And gratitude. For everything. Gratitude for the fact that I've woken up today. I have another opportunity to live a day on this spectacular rock that careens around the sun faster than any of us can imagine. Gratitude for the money that allows me to pay for the groceries. Gratitude for the two legs that carry me through aisle four. For my precious children. My dear, beloved friends. Extended family. Dr. A. The sunshine soaking into my bones. The hot shower. The oat milk lattes that continue to fuel my world (and if you haven't tried them, do yourself a favor and order one—game changer). And gratitude for the fact that I will probably get the chance to do it all again tomorrow. Once we realize just how fleeting and precious life is, somehow what matters comes into very sharp focus, like a telescope requiring the smallest adjustment. At forty-five, I now see so very clearly the beauty, the pain, and the exquisite joy that surrounds us at every turn, if we only just adjust our focus. And then what matters is suddenly perfectly clear.

Of course, it wasn't always so. At twenty-five, I was awash with insecurities. A passive-aggressive comment from my new in-laws would send me reeling, spiraling into my own angst.

Rage internalized at the offense. Fast forward twenty years, and we have a wonderful relationship. I love them more than Brian! (My running joke.) They're wonderful, kind people, and I'm also pretty sure that I'm Cheryl's favorite ex-daughter-in-law. Having said that, I'm her only daughter-in-law, ex or otherwise. But here's the thing: It doesn't matter. None of it matters. Sure, the hurtful comments cut to my core in my youth. Older and wiser now, I see that these were her issues and insecurities projected onto her new daughter-in-law.

And the response now to a hurtful comment, from anyone? Well, it's love. Compassion. Kindness. Think about it. What we are witnessing is another human in pain, and when they don't know what to do with this pain, it's projected outward, onto the closest human in the vicinity. And what does this person need? Kindness. That's what. And kindness is contagious, quite the added bonus! There's a definite ripple effect.

Many of us will spend a lifetime in the future or the past, and in doing so miss the majority of our lives. How incredibly sad. Life is brief! Do we really want to spend that time ruminating about what Auntie Whoever said last week? Or a cruelty inflicted twenty years ago? Perhaps alternating between regrets from the past and fears for the future. Wonderful! Now let's invest the remainder of our precious energy into worrying about events that are largely out of our control! If it sounds unhealthy, it is. Fortunately, there is an antidote. And it's called the present. Mindfully living in the present to be precise, and I shall continue to strive to spend more of this precious lifetime in the present.

The fresh white linen was cool upon my bed, and a welcome respite from another busy day. While attempting to mindfully relax, I no sooner had rested my head upon my overpriced pillow when I heard my children shout. Decidedly not helping my impending slumber (or mindfulness practice), I sighed.

"Alex! Fuck off!"

"Go to hell, Emily."

"Mummmmyyyyyyyyy!"

Another sigh, and I was up. Naively, I thought the sleep disturbances would end much like the elementary school run and recorder practice (how did any of us survive that?!). But no! It turns out that one's teens are equally successful at disturbing their parents' slumber. At least, mine were.

"Right!" I shouted, equal parts anger and frustration, too tired for my calm, grown-up Mummy voice.

Now while I do maintain that when everyone is shouting, there are no adults left in the room, now was not the time to embrace this wisdom. I was tired, I had an early start the next day, and right now my teenage children were arguing over a pillow. A *pillow*. (Did they need mine?) I wish I was kidding.

"Listen up!" More shouting (mine again). "If you two don't get into bed right now, stop with this disgusting language, and begin to show kindness to each other, you will be getting nothing this Christmas except for a T-shirt. And do you know what this T-shirt will read?!"

I was on a roll now. Their eyes stared at me. Silence, finally.

"*Be. Kind.* That's it. And if this nonsense doesn't end, I'll be having them printed next week." My eyes met theirs with a steely determination to put an end to this bickering (and I was very aware that my calm, mindful demeaner just flew out the window). "Just try me," I challenged them.

More staring, and then Emily spoke. "Mummy, can you please lower your voice? You're going to wake the neighbors."

Too tired to care, I headed back to bed.

botox

Happiness can exist only in acceptance.

—George Orwell

Wrinkles. Acceptance.

Time really does march on, and my face is living proof of that. After making peace with my body, my weight, and my thighs, I realized that true acceptance means accepting all of it. The laugh lines, my expressive forehead, my skin that reveals a childhood outdoors without so much as an ozone layer to protect myself from the harsh Australian sun.

"Oh, a bit of color is good for you. You'll be fine!" My mother's words then, and possibly still now. A different generation, I know. They didn't have mineral sunscreens, chemical sunscreens, invisible sunscreens . . . talk about decision fatigue. The process of shopping for sunscreens is almost as overwhelming as my sun-damaged skin.

Acceptance. I keep coming back to this word. And so much more than a phrase, radical acceptance has truly transformed my life (thank you, Tara Brach). The time has come to own my goddamn wrinkles. My changing body. My faded stretch marks. They bear witness to a half a lifetime truly lived.

I am resisting Botox. Full disclosure, I tried it once—just my forehead, and I hated it. I suddenly couldn't move my eyebrows properly. I was frozen! And honestly, when I tried to raise my eyebrows, I looked bloody weird! It was horrible. I spent the next three months trying desperately (in vain) to bring the wrinkles back. Every day in the mirror I'd attempt to contort my forehead, willing the Botox to dissipate, reasoning that with my iron-clad will, anything was possible. Well, it turns out that Botox really does work. Much to my chagrin, I was unable to move a damn thing, and I missed my face. I missed being able to widen my eyes in moments of incredulity (which, in my world, happened daily). I no longer looked like myself. And of course, the children didn't know, until they did.

One day in the kitchen I was trying to explain something, and Emily exclaimed, "Oh my God, Mummy, what is with your *face*? Your eyebrows! They look super creepy!"

"What?" I ask, feigning curiosity—and likely failing at that as I couldn't move anything above my eyeballs.

"*Aaaahhhhh!* Don't do it. That's freaking me out!"

No kidding. You and me both, kid.

I was trying to express emotion, and alas, wound up looking like my eyebrows had some kind of ministroke. The response from my seventeen-year-old was telling. Why is it that an older man looks more distinguished with lines on his face, and as women we are considered less so?

My children laughed for a good three days over Mummy's weird eyebrows and frozen forehead. As for me, it was one and done. Never again, reasoning that I'd just have to find a better night cream.

Kate Winslet, a personal hero of mine for her passionate views, has been vocal in her desire to age gracefully, despite the insane pressures from Hollywood. Thank you, Kate. Having also struggled under the spotlight with her weight, I've always found her relatable. And how grateful was I not to have the battle with my weight documented so publicly, and from such a vulnerable young age. I only had to contend with my mother-in-law and her rude friends. Well, and the strangers.

One particular stranger I'll never forget. I walked into the same posh store in my neighborhood, several years apart. Same saleslady, different treatment. First visit: I was overweight and frumpily dressed. She was overtly rude to me, and her look spoke volumes. "You don't belong here." Ugh. The look of personal offense at my overweight existence I will never forget. Seriously, you'd think I'd walked in with some kind of vile stench following me, such was the intensity of her disdain.

Second visit: I was slim and well-dressed. Of course, I'd just been to the hairdressers, so I was reasonably well put together on this pleasant spring morning. This same lady couldn't have been more welcoming. Falling over herself to help me and successfully part me with my limited funds. How ironic that on my first visit, I had far more money to freely spend and was far less welcome.

It's just so very sad, isn't it? Was my money a different color that day? Was I any less worthy as a human being when I was overweight? No, I bloody well wasn't! The men were just as bad. And it's disgusting. Not all of them, but some were visibly rude to me, as if my extra kilos were distressing to their eyes—I was somehow offending them with my presence. I find myself in a strange predicament today. I now have the kind of figure that men appreciate, and I am treated accordingly. Most men will bend over backward to be helpful when I smile. I smiled when I was fat too, but it didn't hold the same power. Psychology tells us that on some very deep level, all men are thinking, *I might have sex with her one day.* They all want to procreate with someone that they are physically attracted to on a deep, primal level, even if the possibility is nil in the real world. Survival of the species and all that.

Do I enjoy male attention now that I am, in their eyes, suitable mating material? Yes, I do—when it's desired. Of course, I won't lie. Have I forgotten the treatment that I received by many in society when I was overweight and deemed somehow less worthy? No, I haven't.

But do you know what I enjoy far more than positive male attention? Feeling strong. Feeling fit. Energized when I wake. Confident. Comfortable in my clothes. Comfortable in an economy airline seat. Priceless. Now living my own personal MasterCard ad.

As I continue to grow and mature, I care less and less about what men may or may not think about my physical appearance. Fuck it. Sure, I have the bloated PMS days and I'm self-conscious, but then I remember . . . acceptance. First and foremost, I want to look good for me. Feel good for me. Energized from within. And when we feel good internally, it's reflected externally.

I'm also beginning to question my role in society as a woman. How do I want to show up in this next stage of my life? In my relationships? As a mother and role model for my children? I know that I want to show up with kindness, for myself and others, and with confidence . . . respectful, humble confidence. And with power. The power to ask for what I want, to go after what I want. To not apologize for who I am. Ever. For my thighs. My thoughts. My wrinkles.

The patriarchy taught me to be less than, submissive. What does he need? What does he want? How can I bend myself, mold myself to his desires? And it was all unconscious, for the longest time. Society taught us this. Good girls don't argue, they don't speak up. Well, I'm done. We're allowed to speak up, to be angry. And why is an angry woman labeled "difficult" yet an angry man "assertive"?

Remain small, smile, laugh, but don't laugh too loudly. Grandmother wouldn't approve of that either. Well, fuck them all. And if I cook for a man now, it's because I want to. It's out of love, not some inane need for approval or antiquated gender roles, and it's reciprocated with acts of love and kindness from him. Anything less simply won't be tolerated. I'm just too old to put up with any man's shit at this point in my life. Actually, anyone's shit.

move

Walking is the best possible exercise.
Habituate yourself to walk very far.

—Thomas Jefferson

Everything changes when you're slim. Everything. The world is a kinder place.

"Excuse me, excuse me." I delicately tried to wake the man seated next to me. *This is the last time I'll book a window seat*, I mused. Flying economy is unpleasant enough, but with sciatica pain, a full bladder, and two tall men sleeping to my left, I was trapped. While looking grumpy at being awakened, I flashed my brightest smile, murmuring "Thank you!" and the man smiled back, softening.

The world is friendlier.

About fifteen years ago, and in a similar situation, I was seated next to a petite woman in her twenties. I'll never forget the look of disappointment when she realized that she was seated next to me. Was she allergic to fat people? Was she worried that by some process of osmosis she was in danger of gaining weight? My existence seemed to personally offend her. I recall trying to make myself smaller, not daring to share the armrest for risk of offending her further. I should probably point out that while I never did need a seatbelt extender on a flight, I probably came close.

The sciatica pain started a few years ago. "Wear and tear" was Dr. A's explanation. Mileage. Too much weight carried for too long I suspect, and he didn't know this yet. I wasn't ready to tell him. The last remaining legacy of my disordered eating. Shame. And being bloody uncomfortable on long-haul flights. Ironic that my derriere—now one of my favorite body parts—is the one to cause me pain. The universe definitely has a sense of humor, of this I am certain.

Everything is easier now. Maneuvering in and out of an economy airline seat. Running upstairs, receiving help. The world smiles at me now. I'm deemed acceptable. Worthy. Welcome. And it's not okay. For the longest time, I've been watching from the sidelines, following the conversation of weight with interest. Mine is a unique position to be in, and I no longer wish to be silent. It is time to enter the conversation.

Statistically, most people who gain and lose the kind of weight that I did invariably regain it all within the first five years. Many within the first year. I am an anomaly, an outlier. Yet another reason that I wish to share my story, despite the fear of rejection and exposure that I have deliberately avoided in my new world. Appropriate that North America was once the New World, as for me this is exactly what it has been. My new world. The next chapter in my story. After a decade of health, ten years of keeping the weight off, I now know that I will maintain my health for life. I have no doubt. I am simply not the same anxious young girl that I once was. The girl who wanted desperately to be loved, to be accepted, and found a substitute for love in the refrigerator.

Ram Dass told us that it will be enough when it's enough. He spoke of overeating in his seminal work, *Be Here Now*, and he was right. It's 6:00 a.m., and as I watch the sky turn a pale blue over the spectacular Wyoming mountains, I realize that it is enough. My body is truly experiencing a peace and calm that I didn't know possible. I have made peace with my body, my hungers, my desires. I eat when I'm hungry and don't when I'm not. I honor my body's wishes.

When we truly live *in* the body, we're able to access an inner calm and stay grounded. An inherent wisdom. We are all born with it. Five-year-old Jane certainly had it. She didn't head to the refrigerator when she was sad in an attempt to escape her feelings. That had yet to be learned. And unlearned. And we can all unlearn it.

Exercise has been integral to the ongoing maintenance of my health this past decade. Fortunately, I have discovered a true passion for movement in so many forms. Hiking, mountain biking, skiing, yoga, walking. "Exercise puts life into our time." Who said that? Someone wise. My therapy time, hiking leaves me energized, elated with that endorphin high that all athletes know well. My world feels all wrong without movement. After all, we are meant to move. Our bodies are not meant to sit all day. Of this, I am sure.

Life has become far too easy now, as many of us realize. Minimal energy expenditure—maximum energy consumed. I hack my day, walking to buy the daily bread and so forth. These small acts ensure that my body is happy—I'm expending energy and enjoying movement. These incremental changes, made with awareness, have assisted in maintaining my weight loss. Yes, I'm human. Sure, I'll crave cookies. And when I do, I may bake them. Or the craving may pass. Essential is that moment of pause. I'll check in and ask myself, *What am I hungry for? Is it truly the chocolate chip cookie? Sometimes yes. Or is it avoidance? Am I avoiding paperwork?*

That difficult phone call. The twenty-three errands that always find their way to my to-do list?

Red wine and cheese on a Friday evening—still one of my favorite things! (Well, the lactose-free cheeses these days, let's be clear—we don't need another *albergue* washroom-in-Europe debacle). I'll indulge and enjoy this occasionally, but ever mindful of balance.

For the longest time I wished to leave the past behind, escaping from times I'd sooner forget. And then it dawned upon me: Every event, good or bad, significant or otherwise, has led me here and made me who I am. Would I have the compassion for my clients that I have had I not lived some of their pain? My experience growing up with a largely absent parent and family dysfunction, my own separation and divorce, and parenting three wonderful children—one autistic and nonbinary—are life experiences that I'm able to bring into my sessions with clients—invaluable. A disclaimer: I am by no means implying that firsthand experience is necessary to be an effective therapist. I can only speak for myself when I say that my personal growth and life experience has allowed me to step into the role of counselor with a far deeper understanding of the human condition. And in a world that idolizes youth, I am grateful for my career that privileges life experience, where advanced age is seen as an advantage, not a disadvantage. Where corporations will push people at a certain age into retirement, these same executives will likely be looking for a therapist with maturity—gray hair equated with wisdom.

Will I be ready to embrace gray hair when that day arrives in totality? It's a good question. For now, a few gray hairs are concealed by my wonderful hairdresser and her semipermanent-looks-like-my-own-brunette shade of magic, and God bless her. I can't deny feeling that it may take a while before I'm ready to radically accept this life change!

the portal

To travel is to live.

—Hans Christian Anderson

Another airport. Another delay. Flying is waiting, again. The portal, my home away from home, connecting together the pieces of my world with bad food, queues, and flying metal tubes outfitted with row after row of uncomfortable seating, facilitating movement from one world into the next. The challenge in the portal, and elsewhere, is staying grounded within myself while the world spins ever faster. Meditation helps—when I remember to practice. (Still working on this one . . .)

A few stolen moments of sleep and one world recedes into the background, replaced with the next. And my heart, what of that? A piece in Australia with my mother and sister. The largest piece with my children in Vancouver. Kellie, also half a world away. Dr. A in Wyoming. Scattered pieces, belonging to others still, in other corners of the world. It's a curious thing, this feeling of my heart in many places at once. How is this possible? Mine is something of a global existence these days. Long hours spent in the portal, my airport conduit from one world to the next.

"Life is either a daring adventure or nothing." Helen Keller was correct. For me, there was never a choice—mine would be a daring adventure!

"Oh, Janey, you've always been a dreamer!" shared Helen Edwards from next door, many years ago, affectionately shaking her head at me—as if this was something of a charming flaw in my character. I now see that this was the greatest of compliments. Who the hell wouldn't want to be a dreamer?! I know one thing for sure: If I wasn't a dreamer, my life would look very different today. I witness people in my life that say no instead of yes, doubting their abilities, decisions driven by fear. Doubt has no place in my new world, nor fear.

I do my best to pass the time, amusing myself in the portal with people watching (and ever on the lookout for FF nominees). Possibly even more fun has been the watching of my luggage, made possible by the genius that is the AirTag. And fun fact! Your luggage doesn't always travel on the same flight as you, no matter what the airlines say. AirTags don't lie! How do I know this? Because one sunny winter's day, my checked bag arrived in Jackson Hole a good four hours before I did.

"Why didn't we put you on that flight?!" asked a perplexed Dr. A.

How should I know? All I know is that my scuffed white suitcase was patiently waiting for my arrival near the oversized bag collection area (and to be clear, it wasn't oversized! I hate to check a bag, but ski gear necessitated a checked bag this time). And I learned something new that day: our bags don't always stay with us. The upshot of all of this is that I now have a new hobby. Tracking my luggage has become a curious way to pass the time when flying. When that fails, I track my offspring. It's brilliant. In a couple of seconds, I can see exactly where my three children are on the planet, with surprising accuracy.

My mother has also taken to tracking my whereabouts with stalker-like vigilance. She loves it, and I suppose as she nears seventy, it is a viable hobby. I'm convinced it's become a game for Jan as she tracks my iPhone (thank you, Family Sharing). No sooner would I land somewhere or arrive home from the supermarket and be making my way to the bathroom, I would receive an enthusiastic "Welcome home!" from mother. Secretly, I think it's lovely. My kids are less excited about being tracked 24-7, but frankly, there are what, eight billion of us now on this overcrowded planet? I prefer to go to bed at night knowing where my three offspring are.

Finally, I boarded, another delay over. And in the infinite wisdom that was this airline, they seated two octogenarians in the exit rows in front of me and just asked them if they could operate the doors in the case of an emergency landing. I'd like to stress the following here: They couldn't even hear the question being asked! As for pushing open a forty-plus pound emergency door, I wished them good luck. God help us all.

Pretty sure if this plane goes down, we're all done for. And I certainly don't mean to appear ageist in my assessment of this situation, but it did seem to me that the airline could have allocated those seats to more able passengers!

Was flying always this unpleasant? The man in front and diagonally opposite was in danger of hacking up a lung. Possibly both. He mercifully donned a mask, only to remove it to eat his packed lunch. Hacking continued. If we didn't die when the elderly people failed to assist us in an emergency, I was quite sure we'd all die after contracting whatever disease this unwell man was transmitting to every man, woman, and child on board. *Give me strength.*

"Aaahhhhhkkkk-ugh." The hacking cough continued. I decided to say another prayer. It couldn't hurt.

And why is it that every airline on Earth feels the need to blast their cabins with refrigerator-cold air? Is it a distraction technique? Perhaps an attempt to distract from the inedible food and uncomfortable seats at the back of the plane? The mind boggles. So many questions. I've taken to traveling with my own wool blanket, eye mask, and memory foam neck pillow. For me the only way if attempting to achieve any measure of sleep. I do remain grateful to have the means to travel and recognize that this is a luxury not afforded to all. I'll also admit that I'm still working on acceptance as it relates to flying. The terminals, the queues, the delays . . . it's just not one of my favorite things. I do also recognize that airlines need to make a profit, and that the aviation industry is likely doing the best it can to move millions of us around the globe safely, year after year, and for that I remain grateful.

Home is my sanctuary, despite my wanderlust. Controlling nutrition is far easier in my own kitchen. Travel in the States, not so much. The portions are enormous, the food largely processed, a random assortment of sugar, oil, and flour. It's really quite revolting. More than once I've found myself looking at a menu and not finding one thing that I actually want to put into my body. This doesn't apply to high-end restaurants, where the food is usually excellent. It's a constant challenge to find unprocessed food in the land of mass-processed crap. Also something of a challenge in the portal. Of course, my dear svelte friend Charlotte says, "Oh, Jane, just grab a glass of wine or two. That's what I do whenever I fly!" Easy for her to say. Charlotte has been wearing the same size jeans since I've met her and, for some inexplicable reason, seems incapable of converting alcohol calories to fat cells. My constitution is quite the opposite.

Mine is a constant challenge to keep my weight within certain acceptable numbers on the scale (to be clear—acceptable for me, not society), and more than that, ensuring my pants still do up. Ensuring that I wake every day with energy and vigor as time marches on.

Now I love a good gin and tonic in summer more than most, but given that my body excitedly stores any excess energy with the efficiency of the North Korean army, moderation is my friend. Well, that and periods of abstinence. A month without alcohol does wonders for keeping my weight in check.

Moderation.

My weight has certainly fluctuated over the years, a few pounds up and down. I suspect that this is common for most of us as the seasons change. I mean, who doesn't eat a little too much in December?!

Looking back, I can easily equate periods of daily walking with periods of health in my pre-baby days. Nowadays walking is a daily constant, nonnegotiable, and a joy. Perhaps I was always seeking . . . the walking a metaphor for my search. This yearning for meaning, for purpose, for love, for answers. And I walk fast, I always have. I was always moving, searching, unsure of the destination but certain that I was destined for somewhere else (and as far away from Broken Hill as possible). I should probably stress that some people love Broken Hill, it's just not for everybody. Much like Nebraska, Broken Hill just wasn't for me. Can you believe this was, until very recently, Nebraska's official tourism slogan?! Seriously, it read as follows: "Nebraska. Honestly, it's not for everyone." Mind you, perhaps Broken Hill should consider adopting the same.

"Routines are for idiots!" declared Kellie's mother some years back. I tended to take Gloria's advice with a grain of salt, given that she also felt that bras, dinner plates, and cutlery were unnecessary for the most part. Gloria raised five children, and I often wonder how that must have worked with her no-routine policy.

As for myself—a somewhat moderate parent—I attempted to implement a flexible routine with my little ones, and it seemed to work for the most part. Routine is also helpful during weight loss and maintenance, otherwise we're all just flying blind. Now I don't know about anyone else, but I imagine that flying blind will likely lead to a plane crash, or in my case, a visit to the local department store to purchase elasticized pants. No, thank you.

Despite declarations of freedom, we humans are creatures of habit. A habit is typically defined as something that is unintentional, uncontrollable, and efficient. We also lack full awareness of engaging in the habit. Formed in roughly four weeks (this is still debated), and in my experience faster still to fall by the wayside. Without question, continued commitment to these healthy habits is my portal to health, to wellness, to thriving.

Clearly, healthy habit formation has been key in helping to maintain my weight loss. Scientists now know that the brain is malleable, able to be rewired. Neuroplasticity! And thank the Lord for that. Visual reminders, rewards, small acts of self-compassion, meditation, and yoga are among my effective daily strategies to help stay on track. And please don't think that I'm describing denial. Moderation, yes. Balance. I know my body. I know that if I enjoy a twice-baked almond croissant one day, it's best done after a hike, thus preventing the croissant from finding its way to permanently settle onto my ass. No, thank you.

cravings

Between stimulus and response there is a space. In that space is our power to choose our response. In our response lies our growth and our freedom.

—Viktor E. Frankl

I avoided a lot—decades of avoidance, in hindsight. And I'm still working on it. A tough day can still challenge me. Standing at the pantry, jar in hand—or perhaps it was a spoon this time? Hmm . . . what were we craving today? Almonds, granola, dried apricots, dark chocolate? You see, my overeating was often healthy foods, so I fooled myself into thinking that perhaps this was actually good for me and, well, it just wasn't that bad I'd reasoned. (Truthfully, I could probably talk myself into anything.) But the problem wasn't in the food, it was in the cravings, the quantity, the emotional eating. The hunger. And not for food. For escape. It was the *why*. Why was I standing at the pantry, in front of that door? I knew damn well—it was avoidance at play. Avoiding the chores, the to-do list, the mundane crap that every stay-at-home mother knows all too well. The problem was that in these moments, I was avoiding *my life*. A life that I had willingly signed up for. Make no mistake, I have no regrets. But I also had no idea of what was to come—none of us does.

"If she was my first, she would have been the last!" An acquaintance discussed her four daughters, the youngest teen going through something of a difficult stage. I could relate, but for me the horse had already bolted. I was pregnant with my second by Cerulean's first birthday party. My three finest achievements and joys. How could I possibly regret past decisions?

The point I wish to make is that it took many years (and a master's degree in psychology) to realize that this avoidant behavior, this disordered eating, was driven by anxiety. When I'd become overwhelmed by the growing demands on my shoulders, I would seek an escape. Hungry for an escape, mine became the sugar-laden granola. My problem was that I was eating it after a full meal. My body didn't need or want it; my mind did. Hence we had a disconnect, and I needed far better coping mechanisms. After all, my responsibilities weren't going anywhere anytime soon, and as I'm discovering now, they don't magically evaporate when our children become young adults. Sure, they change. Parenting becomes more emotional, less physical. Little people, little problems. Big people, big problems. We are parenting until the day we die, and anybody contemplating parenthood needs to be aware of this responsibility. At least if they wish to do it well.

Stuck in the portal again. My mind turns to food. I'm bored. Tired. And I want my bed. I don't want overpriced airport food. I want to be in my shower, followed closely by my warm bed, clean linen, and welcome solitude. Mindfulness is still work. I remind myself to breathe. Check in. Come home to myself. I slow my breathing and turn inward. My stomach tells me that it's content; it doesn't want food, having eaten an early dinner prior to entering the portal. I practice interoceptive awareness. It's really the easiest thing and the hardest. To be truly present, anchored within ourselves, mindfully in the present, where peace is to be found. Where I can intentionally tune into my body's hunger signals, feel my body's needs. I breathe. Here. Now.

I look around, surveying the terminal as I wait by the departure gate. I notice the elderly lady working on her cross stitch. *Do they allow those needles on flights now?* I wonder. The cute backpacker who has me yearning to pack my own and take that long desired sabbatical (with or without cute, ripped backpacker). The older couple, he in his casual golf course T-shirt, she with the dated '80s hairstyle. Can we please just outlaw anything remotely '80s? Clothing. Music. Hairstyles. Is there anything more disturbing than the '80s? Seriously, I don't care if it's in vogue again and the kids think it's cool. That doesn't make the mullet any less hideous. Good Lord. Living it once was bad enough. Do we need to go there again?!

Ram Dass tells us that it's good to learn to wait. To delay gratification. Air Alaska is ensuring that my gratifying shower is delayed, and so I wait in the portal, attempting to be present. Every opportunity a chance to practice mindfulness. Like a small child learning to ride a bike, I practice. Because, the thing is, when we to truly listen to our bodies, they will invariably tell us what we need. Whenever my actions align with my body's needs, I feel a deep calm. My body thanks me for respecting its wishes. After all, when we eat out of boredom or because our flight is delayed and we're stuck, respect for our bodies goes out the window.

After several decades, I'm finally respecting my body's wishes, finally in alignment with my own needs. And it's a gamechanger. But it's not always easy. I frequently remind myself to come back to my body, to turn inward, and reconnect with myself. A constant practice, and like a muscle at the gym, when we exercise it, it gets stronger. My body says, "Thank you." I'm sitting on the plane. Tired, yet proud of my growth. I resisted the mindless eating to pass the time. And I realize just how far I've come. And I also realize that, through the practice of mindfulness, I truly feel myself in this body now. Embodiment. My weight on the aircraft seat. My feet on the floor, my legs sink into the chair, my spine pressing into the back of the seat. And my internal voice gets louder. And clearer. It's about 9:00 p.m. as we finally take to the skies.

I'll eat breakfast tomorrow. I'm not physically hungry now. I'm hungry for a shower. For my bed.

And I listen. It's nothing short of a revelation. I realize that I was so disconnected from my body for so many years, I couldn't even begin to hear that voice. If I did, it was ignored. Why? Was it comfort I needed? Was that what food provided? Certainly, at times. I escaped, avoiding everything. Avoiding life.

And the answer now? I can comfort myself. I am whole. Complete. And grateful. And no longer needing or wanting to escape. And here's the thing: *We need to build a life that we don't want to escape from!*

I am convinced that gratitude is the answer—to everything. If only I could go back and tell my twenty-year-old self this, but life doesn't work this way, and for a reason! We need to *learn* these lessons! There's simply no substitute for life experience. I see that now.

patriarchy

*If patriarchy had a specific beginning
in history, it can also have an end.*

—Maria Mies

Fuck the patriarchy. I bought the keychain. I bought my daughter the keychain. Taylor Swift is right, and if there's a single message that a young woman in 2023 needs to hear and remember more than this one, I am yet to find it.

Our children watch us. They learn from us and take their cues from our actions, for better or worse. When I left Brian, he told me that the children would ask questions one day, hold me accountable for the divorce. And perhaps they will, but they will also see a woman who made decisions that were brave and not driven by fear. Fear immobilizes; it keeps us safe. I could have stayed. I had financial security. A credit card to use freely (within reason). I didn't have to work outside the home. To the outside world, my decisions may not have made a lot of sense, but my concern was not for the outside world and their never-ending judgments. My concern was for my soul.

As I ponder my relationship with Dr. A, I am struck by some rather patriarchal realities. You see, Dr. A, being eleven-and-a-half years my senior, was born into a slightly different world. And fun fact—curiously my former Latin lover was eleven-and-a-half years my junior. Surely the gods knew of this when our worlds collided that day in the elevator.

Despite only joking to confirm the following, I'm aware that he does indeed appreciate my presence in his kitchen, barefoot and compliant. Now while I do love to be both barefoot and in my own kitchen, I enjoy the experience most when it's of my own volition. The expectation as the one in the relationship with the XX chromosomes, and therefore the one more often in the kitchen, doesn't sit well with me. To be fair, I have more free time, and I love to cook. It's the implications that remain problematic. We fall into these gendered relationship roles so very easily, and once patterns become established, it feels harder to extricate oneself from the assumed role. I remain conflicted.

Will our story have a happy ending? I can no sooner predict this than I can predict the direction of the wind tomorrow. What I do know is that my new relationship looks very different from past ones. Perhaps I sound like a man hater—I'm not. Dr. A is a good man, but I know in this relationship what I will and won't accept. And I will give all of myself willingly, but I know my worth, what I'll tolerate. Life is just too short for anything less.

As I write this, I near my forty-sixth birthday, and I know that if I'm extremely lucky I may have another forty-six summers. Another forty-six winters, cozy by the fire and curled up with a good book, and it dawns on me—this really isn't very long. After all, the last forty-six have gone by in a blink. What do I want the next forty-six to look like? The stoic philosopher Seneca tells us that life is long enough when well-lived, when used wisely. I aim to remember this, embrace this wisdom, and allow it to guide my decisions henceforth.

"You know, my kids will probably dump me in a nursing home when I'm old . . ." Dr. A mused in bed.

"Well, if I stick around, I won't let that happen. Not to worry!" I joked.

"Aww . . . you'll take care of me?" he asked and smiled.

"No, I'll hire a nurse!"

It was my turn to smile. Problem solved.

Of course, this conversation took us both decades into a potential future, and not one that either of us is ready to ponder. I know I'm certainly not. I've only just obtained my freedom after decades with the same man, as a wife and mother. Do I ever want to give that up? Ever?

No, I don't. Certainly not yet, anyway.

Thunder. The air was clean and cool after the afternoon cloud burst. I'd been watching the clouds build all morning over the mountains to the west, hopeful, anticipating a storm reminiscent of the Australian outback thunderstorms of my childhood. Then Dr. A and I found ourselves in bed. Something of a regular occurrence when together, given the nature of our long-distance relationship. And seriously, if there's a better place to be during a thunderstorm than between clean sheets with one's lover, I'm yet to find it.

Thunder and lightning. Two of my favorite things! Along with lattes, Latin lovers, live music, hot showers, sleeping outdoors, a good book, and pretty dresses. Now, despite my father's assertion that the world can be divided into animal lovers or not, I also believe that the world can be divided into those who love lightning and those who fear it. I imagine it tells us a little something about personality types. Having said that, I've never been hit by lightning. Perhaps I'd be a little less excited about a storm if I was one of the unfortunate people to have been struck down by an angry thunderbolt from the gods. The world is new and fresh, the air delicious after the storm—still one of my favorite scents.

The pillow-talk turned to our mutual online dating horror stories.

"I once had a first date with a city bus driver," I told Dr. A. "It's an honest living, and I absolutely reserved judgment about his vocation. But here's the thing. . . . Five minutes into the conversation it became clear that he wasn't a closet philosopher . . . or any type of philosopher."

Dr. A. chuckled. He'd had his share of dating nightmares. The unresolved traumas, the angry exes, the functional alcoholics, the workaholics—often all rolled into one. And God bless men, the visual creatures that they are. Many men will overlook the red flags if she's hot enough. Fuckable enough. Am I wrong?

"Why did you agree to drinks?" he asked.

"I like drinks!" I kidded, playful. But truthfully, it was clear that while Mr. Bus Driver didn't read Nietzsche in his spare time, he must have spent an inordinate amount of time at the gym, such was the physique under his shirt. And I did appreciate the effort that he put in to don a collared shirt. That was sweet. He also had one of those heavenly symmetrical faces with, what mother would call bedroom eyes, plus a gorgeous smile. Our waitress certainly noticed that evening when she brazenly left her number with a heart on the bill. (Can you believe that? In front of me!)

"Look, he was a gentleman, but it became clear very quickly that the conversation was lacking."

"Ahh." Dr. A nodded.

"I do appreciate that you're a doctor, I won't pretend otherwise. I mean, there's a feeling of safety that comes with knowing that when we're out to dinner, if I choke on something, you'll probably be able to save my life. I mean, you'll certainly know what to do. With the bus driver, I'm a sitting duck!"

"Well, he'd get you to the hospital," mused Dr. A. "He'd just make a few stops along the way . . ." Dr. A chuckled.

"Yes, yes, he would." I stretched out, also laughing, and said a quick prayer of thanks, grateful that I no longer endure random first dates with hot men who drive buses.

marriage

Look closely at the present you are constructing:
it should look like the future you are dreaming.

—Alice Walker

"Well, she's your problem now, Brian!" my mother jested, the scene my long-ago wedding reception. Said lightly, but it spoke to something much larger than the state of my thighs. Why is a married daughter considered offloaded, suddenly a burden released? Was I a burden? I suppose I did spend an inordinate amount of time in the kitchen whenever I'd visit home, so Jan could have argued that her grocery bill was now lower. Well, so are my expectations of men nowadays. After all, expectation is the root of all heartache.

Marriage just doesn't sit well with me these days. The whole antiquated concept of "Here, please take my daughter, three cows, and a goat." I realize that I've come full circle, from the enthusiastic young girl who wanted the white wedding, to the girl who felt incomplete without a boyfriend, to the woman who actively opposes any type of formal union with anyone. Fiercely independent and not wishing to ever answer to anyone again, about anything, I've fought too hard for my independence to give it up again. And anyway, I'm pretty sure my dad's all out of goats.

"Well, Jane, you know, a husband would be useful . . ."
my mother declared, postdivorce, pondering my prospects,
Jane Austen-style. I remain to be convinced. After all, what I
really wanted was my freedom—my autonomy—and I have
that now! And you can't put a price on freedom. Mind you,
Brad would disagree. He's a criminal defense attorney.

Anyway, what on Earth would I do with a husband?!
Not to mention the fact that married men live longer than
their unmarried counterparts. Married women do not. That's
right. A married woman is statistically more likely to die
younger than her single friends. Now if that isn't an argument
for rejecting matrimony, then I don't know what is. Why any
woman would wish to remarry after learning of this statistic
is beyond me. Or marry in the first place. The lure of an early
death?! A hard pass for me if ever there was one. I love life,
and I'd like to continue to live it for as long as possible.

Marriage is an exercise in optimism, and I've decided
that even for a wildly optimistic person such as myself, still
a stretch. I'd like to tell you that the story of myself and Dr. A
ends with us sailing off into the sunset, our tale neatly wrapped
in a red bow. Perhaps it will, but life rarely works out like that.
I've learned over the years that the least likely and most unpredictable thing will invariably happen. I've also learned that life
has a beautiful way of unfolding just as it's meant to. As I grow
and evolve, I've come to realize that, at forty-five, I don't wish
to be legally tethered or bound to any man.

Perhaps I've always been a free spirit at heart, yearning
to be set loose to explore foreign shores. Some find comfort
in consistency, security, and keeping their worlds small. Not
I. I ache to have the freedom to come and go as I please.
Work as a remote counselor would facilitate this (thank you,
pandemic) or as a published writer. I plan to do both—and

explore the world as I do. My children are all but grown, and I'm acutely aware that in two and a half years my youngest child will likely begin university, and my world will suddenly and dramatically change again.

Change. The only constant.

When I decided to write this book and share my humble story, I knew with a certainty in my bones that I was meant to share it, that my next career would be that of author. I love to write! And where will I be one year from now? Five years from now? Backpacking my way through Europe, perhaps? Completing another stage of another Camino? Driving a Sprinter van around this fine continent? God only knows, and frankly, I'd rather be surprised. What I do know is that one year from now, I will be continuing to nurture my body and soul with good food, joyful movement, friendships, love, and oat milk lattes in all their overpriced glory!

Do I ask for too much? Brian would probably say yes. But can any of us ask for too much out of life? And who defines too much? Society? The church?

"You're aggressive," Sebastian told me once, years back.

"Well, how else do I get what I want?" I asked him. "I won't apologize for that."

He looked over, thoughtful, respecting my honesty.

Most men don't like aggressive though; I learned that lesson years ago. They also don't want things to be too easy. There's a logic behind these ridiculous games that we all play. During any courtship, it is well known that a woman is considered more desirable when she is less attainable, less available. She will invariably turn down an invitation in order to allow the pursuer to continue to pursue.

"Treat 'em mean, keep 'em keen!" Auntie Sue's wisdom, right again. Men like a challenge, the hunt. The chase. I'm convinced that this is a direct result of evolution. They're hardwired to hunt, pursuing the wild animal that will be dinner for the clan. Men don't want a woman to make herself too available, too easy to conquer any more than they would want the animal in the wild to lie down at their feet, waiting for death. Where's the challenge in that?!

Take my dear Brad, for example. He shared his story over yet another excellent bottle of red from his wine room. What can I say? I do consider it my civic duty to help him drink it. (Frankly, it's like community service.) As I sunk into his oversized sofa, glass in hand, he began to explain his latest girlfriend dilemma.

"It's too easy now, Janey. There's no challenge! She doesn't make me work for anything."

And in this confession, I was given a window into the secret life of the heterosexual male brain (at least Brad's). Nothing if not interesting, I listened.

"In the beginning I had to work for it! Seriously. We had about ten dates before she'd have sex with me," he confided.

"And you respected her more for it," I inferred.

"Of course." Brad's frustration was evident at the time, let me tell you, but it earned the woman in question his respect.

Fast forward six months and where is he now emotionally? Bored, that's where. Now I appreciate that not all men would share this boredom. Brad now has an intelligent, kind woman with whom to share his days. I mean, the woman cleans for him! (Why, I have no idea, yet the fantasy of many a heterosexual male I'm sure, at least when the housekeeper's off duty.) So why is he unhappy? Restless? After all, isn't this what many men dream of? Good, regular sex and a woman who wipes down the countertops. Am I wrong? And why is he restless? Because the chase is over. History tells me that this union will soon end; Brad is restless. What will follow is a three-month Tinder bender of hedonism, followed by another six-month relationship that will end predictably, in much the same way that they all do.

"All men want a lady in public and a whore in the bedroom," I concluded, sharing my opinion over my second glass of excellent pinot.

"Not me," declared Brad. "I want a whore everywhere."

As I write this, all I can think is, *I'm sure as hell not going to be wiping some man's countertops or smiling sweetly as I sweep his floors in some insane quest for approval like Brad's more domestic-minded girlfriends.* But here's the thing: I do appreciate a clean house. I don't wish to live surrounded by crap any more than I'm willing to deal with other people's. Hence, I'll wipe and sweep and scrub when the need arises. I don't love cleaning, but I'll get it done. It's the why behind the action, not the action itself that I take exception to, in a man's home. The patriarchy really does have a lot to answer for, doesn't it? And anyway, I'm tired of cleaning up other people's crap.

As I write this, my eldest nears their twentieth birthday. I've been cleaning up after a family for two decades. That's a bloody long time. No wonder I want to backpack through Europe. While my peers were backpacking across the globe in their twenties, I was cleaning highchairs and preparing organic baby food—of course the firstborn had only the best. By the second, the bar was somewhat lower. And by the third, my firstborn was something of a challenge to parent. Screaming meltdowns were a very regular occurrence.

No one knew why. The handmade, organic baby food sure as hell didn't fix those.

Am I going to have a screaming meltdown of my own? No. Those, too, belong to the past, to the girl who was overwhelmed with responsibility and sought comfort in the refrigerator. I won't melt down, but I will advocate for myself. I'll honor my needs and desires. And when I clean Dr. A's countertops, it's because I wish to work as a team as we cohabitate from time to time. Not because I feel it's expected. But is it? Does he expect it on some level? After all, his workday is far longer than mine. Would he be happy to return after a long day to a messy kitchen? Would I?! I remain conflicted . . . so many unanswered questions.

Blue jobs and pink jobs—that's what my friend Kate calls them. I realize that this language is harmful and exclusionary to my nonbinary eldest (apologies, C.B.). Kate is one half of one of those rare, elusive unions: the happy long-term marriage. She's made it very clear that she and her husband have very defined pink and blue jobs within the marriage, and it works for them. I respect that. They have a mutually agreed division of labor. Do Dr. A and I? After all, he pumps the tires in my bike and oils the chain. He pumps the petrol into the car. And I'm grateful for both (two blue jobs, if ever there were any). Besides, the petrol stinks. I've always hated that smell. The one saving grace of Broken Hill was the kid who would pump the petrol, day in and day out. My hands stayed clean and free of that God-awful smell. So, it wasn't all bad, shithole of a town that it was.

Given that marriage is inherently patriarchal, and not being at all fond of the patriarchy at this point in my life, I'd rather not participate in one of its most oppressive customs. Ever. Does any woman need a husband in 2024? Certainly not in Canada. Historically, marriage ensured that women remained the property of men, subordinate and bound. The questions of inheritance and lineage were ensured. The thing is, I neither wish to own or be owned. As for being subordinate, that's a seriously hard pass. I think I've always been a free soul. I don't think anyone could tie me down at this point if they wanted to.

And that's the curious thing: people will still make antiquated comments regarding my current relationship.

"Oh, you've done well to hold onto him!"

"Don't let this one get away!"

"Oh . . . he's a neurologist!"

Seriously? Hasn't he also done well in securing me as his girlfriend?! What the fuck? Is this 2024 or 1824?!

And there we have it. This underlying and still prevalent view that a woman needs to "catch" a man, secure a good husband. Well, Good Lord.

No. Thank. You.

None of us belongs to another. I belong to me. This rather profound observation occurred while I was alone, hiking. Where else? Reminding me of a young Alexander at age ten, he once declared, "Mummy, I do my best thinking on the creek!" referring to his after-school walk home through nature. And well, Alex, as it turns out, so does Mummy.

So many people experience profound grief when they try in vain to hold onto another person who no longer wants to be held. I think of my Vancouver best friend, Georgia. My dearest friend has navigated possibly the ugliest divorce I think I've ever witnessed. Sadly, at her core, her grief is profound for one reason: She was left for another woman. Her husband chose another, and she was bereft, the grief far deeper due to my friend's attempts (for years) to desperately hold onto this man who no longer wished to be held.

It is entirely fruitless to attempt to hold onto another human being. They don't belong to us. No one does. My children don't belong to me either; they are their own people. Why do we feel ownership over another person?

If someone wishes to enter or remain in my life, I welcome them with love (Tinder sex-pests aside—there are limits). And if someone wishes to leave my world, I let them go with love and wish them well. When did grasping desperately onto someone ever work? In my experience they just pull away and run that much faster, and why wouldn't they? They no longer wish to be there. Let them go!

Years ago, I experienced this firsthand when I had to let go of my eldest child. But what an unexpected gift I received, as Cerulean transitioned into the most wonderful nonbinary child that I've ever had! (And the only one, but let's not get bogged down in the details.) For myself there was a grieving, a letting go of my hopes, dreams, and visions of my child's future. But here's the thing: Those were *my* dreams, not Cerulean's. Their life is not an extension of mine. I can claim no ownership or demands on their future by virtue of being their mother. This life is theirs to live. I think sometimes as parents, we forget this. These are not our lives to live over, vicariously attempting to relive our own, as some parents do.

My child's transition was theirs to make, autonomously. Who are we to tell another human soul how they must feel, act, or dress? Have we inhabited their body? Walked a mile in their hiking boots? No, I bloody well hadn't. And I had to learn this. This realization has allowed me to support my eldest as they navigated some extremely difficult years. The depression Cerulean endured was horrific.

"Perhaps my world seemed so dark to you because your world is so light." Cerulean recently shared this observation, astute as always.

Our children don't belong to us any more than the stars in the sky, both belonging to the universe.

Auntie Sue put it best, warning me many years prior: "Jane, just remember, they're only ever on loan!"

She was correct on that point.

yoga/wine

*If one oversteps the bounds of moderation, the
greatest pleasures cease to please.*

—Epictetus

Geneen Roth passed along tools through her books, and some I use to this day. She tells us that when we're emotional and on the verge of an eating bender, just sit down. Lie down if possible. Rest the body. Pause. And so, I do. My overpriced yoga mat lives almost permanently on my bedroom floor these days for this very reason—and much like a cat, I love to stretch! My reminder. To pause. Stop. Just lie down.

Savasana.

Often, it's exactly what I need. I don't know about you, but my emotions can still overwhelm me at times. I'm just wired this way it seems (and I suspect a lot of us are). My yoga mat has become one of several antidotes. Slowing down invariably helps my mind to calm, where I can begin to process the emotions that have rattled me. A warm bath also helps. I am a water sign after all—Scorpio/Pisces/Scorpio. No wonder I cry so often! And I've always been fond of drawing a bath in the evening—I'm surprised more people don't.

"I don't take baths. I don't get it. Just lying there. Explain it to me," asked my friend Meg, card-carrying member of the First Wives Club. With a wicked sense of humor I do appreciate, she enquired, "What happens in the bath? Seriously, Jane. Do you masturbate? Phone a friend? Tell me. Help me to understand. Candles, music, wine? What's going on in the bath?!"

Our group laughed. Everyone loves Meg for her candid, no-nonsense approach to everything.

"I find it restorative," I told them. "It's very calming, and no, I don't feel the need to masturbate, thank you for asking."

The First Wives Club, of which I am a proud member, consists—as you can probably imagine—of women who are separated and divorced. Some were left, and some did the leaving, and all are bonded over the shared heartbreak that is falling asleep at night with your precious children under a different roof.

Ahh, co-parenting. Not for the faint of heart. I found it got easier as the years passed; for some this hasn't been their experience. Either way we find that wine helps. When doesn't wine help?! (In moderation, of course.) I've long maintained that red wine makes everything better. Well, that and a well-made espresso. In the reverse order.

Possibly the finest example of moderation I've ever witnessed was that of my late Great Auntie Moira. Passing just shy of her ninety-ninth birthday, she denied herself nothing. She walked every day of her life, drank one whisky and water every evening, and maintained a love for life until the very end. Always eating sensible portions of food, she was the very definition of moderation until the day she crossed over from this world to the next. The grandmother I wish I'd had, and my late grandmother's sister, Auntie Moira never failed to make me feel loved; ironically, my late grandmother never succeeded. Did she ever try? Not in my memory.

Now despite my late grandmother's strong feelings on the subject of bananas, I eat a lot of fruit—whole fruit—and I'm pleased to report that it hasn't made me fat again. On the contrary, when I crave something sweet—which is still more often than I'd like—I do find that a piece of fresh fruit increasingly hits the spot. Like any positive habit, the key is repetition. As for fruit juice, I avoid that like online dating apps and juice cleanses—both lead to pain. Best to just stay away. One has way too much sugar, the other has way too many sex pests, and I have no need of either.

When I finished the first draft of this memoir, I stopped drinking. Not forever, just until Christmas, and I'm pleased to report that I've noticed some very immediate benefits! I have more energy, my skin is glowing, and my pants are ever so slightly looser. Win-win-win. Plus—I feel great.

Would I ever give up red wine permanently? Hell no. Will I consider consuming less in the future? Yes. Anyway, Christmas seemed like an appropriate time to break one's period of abstinence. And why have I stopped? After all, I'm by no means a heavy drinker. Because even two glasses of red twice a week was affecting my energy and my skin, and it was beginning to feel just a little harder to maintain my weight within certain numbers that I'm comfortable with. It was time to listen to my body.

Having recently experienced the portal hungover not once but twice, I knew that something had to give. I don't recommend it. Flying economy is insufferable enough. Flying economy with a hangover is nothing short of horrific. Seriously, this could be used as effective punishment for our low-risk criminals! You've committed a white-collar crime? I sentence you to sixty days of economy flying with raging hangovers. Throw in some equally horrific airline food and coffee, and I'm pretty sure they'll think twice before embezzling again.

judgment

Be yourself; everyone else is already taken.

—Oscar Wilde

S nacking was easy, my escape from reality, and I became one hell of a home cook—I still am. The difference between 1994 and 2024 is simple. I now bake when hungry for food, to share food, experimenting with healthy recipes that nurture instead of numb. Cooking became an evolution from the dubious ingredients of my youth to arugula, chia seeds, and almond flour. (In Australia we actually had something called cooking margarine. It was revolting.)

Do I place pressure on myself to maintain this physique? In part yes, and happily so. It's a conscious choice. I won't ever again compromise my health, therefore it's helpful pressure (and quite frankly, I can't afford another new wardrobe of clothes in a bigger size). I'm driven by some very positive factors, being acutely aware that I'm setting an example of health for my kids. Modeling balance. Moderation. And I don't want to die, at least not anytime soon. Lord knows, one of my dear offspring may decide to assist in overpopulating the planet, and if so, I'd like to be here to see it.

But here's the thing: I'm also driven by a desire to stay desirable. Is this a bad thing? Is it wrong to want to look my best? Live my best life, as Kellie would say? So many questions, and the answer: No, it's not. The conflict arises when I feel that pressure coming from a man in the form of judgment, however subtle. It's all tremendously confusing really.

"Are we having toast again?!" A former lover stared at me, incredulous. I was outraged, having prepared a snack after a long day at my crappy, $11-an-hour retail gig.

"Did you just say that?!" My voice was incredulous. I gave him my best Alexander-Paddington Bear hard stare.

And fun fact. This former suitor (and techie) had managed to find what I thought was successfully buried—an elusive photo from my past. Evidently, he stumbled upon this former fat, postbaby photo in the archives of Facebook. Ugh. Clearly my privacy settings needed some tightening—problem solved. So of course, in time he revealed this knowledge of the unearthed photo to me. Ironically, he'd left his unhappy, sexless marriage and a very overweight wife, and God bless him for his honesty.

"Jane, I didn't leave my wife because she was fat. I left her because she didn't clean the house. And I don't want an overweight girlfriend, or she won't have the energy to clean the house either. She'll be too tired for housework!"

"I see." My only response. So very earnest in his assertion. Yet another wonderful example of our thriving patriarchal world.

Thank you. Next.

"Jane, that is the fattest kitten that I have ever seen!"

Now fast forward a decade, and Teddy is likely the fattest cat my mother has ever seen (when we visit them at Brian's home). He is a Big Boy. Having taken to calling him Boofer, my children now accuse me of fat shaming our cat. And perhaps I am. Does my formerly conflicted relationship with food and girth extend to Teddy and Toffee? Possibly. And it's also quite possible that Toffee is afflicted with the same eating disorder that affects many women in Vancouver, because for as much as Teddy is too large, Toffee is too small. Did she get the '90s waif memo too?! Or is it a case of survival of the fittest? Was she not fast enough to her food? I'm still not sure. Either way, I do miss my feline friends. There's definitely a cat in my future. After all—God willing—there's time for me to become a cat lady yet.

"Jane, you still have a lot of guilt around food sometimes."

Perhaps there was some truth to my friend Isabelle's observation (unlike my enormous cat, who shows no sign of concern for his disordered eating).

"Well, after spending the better part of two decades comfort eating, I do think it prudent that perhaps I spend the next few exercising restraint!" I quipped.

I wouldn't say guilt. I would say that I'm conscientious. Balance. I just know how effortlessly my body can gain weight, making new fat cells with wild abandon or plumping up the old ones. I'm something of an expert, and there's a genetic component—my father is living proof of that.

People still ask occasionally, "What did you eat to lose the weight? How did you do it?"

Maintenance is challenging, as many formerly overweight people will tell you. In hindsight, losing weight is the easier part. Momentum begins, and encouraged, success begets success. The adjustment to daily maintenance is a different beast. Suddenly, my new smaller body needed less energy. It's surprising how little food we actually need (and initially, quite depressing). My body also needs to move—daily exercise is essential for my physical and mental health. Quite simply, exercise puts life into my time, and frankly, keeping the weight off is hard work. I've made a commitment to myself to respect my body, to nurture and care for this vessel that will carry me through this lifetime. I do maintain that food must be enjoyed, as one of life's greatest pleasures. The secret is balance.

Internal disorder is reflected externally, of this, I am sure. If I am struggling with eating and with my weight, it is a clear sign that I need to turn inward. That I'm unsettled. Troubled. Every time. What is rattling me? When we cease the behavior of emotional eating, even temporarily, we are forced to look underneath to the root cause, and the driving force is exposed.

I don't think that maintenance ever ends. This need for accountability, to balance my body's energy intake and expenditure as I age hasn't diminished. Curiosity and compassion for my body are essential to my well-being, but there's no escaping the fact that I need to continue to practice moderation daily, unless shopping for pants in a bigger size is something that I'm okay with. And it's not.

I absolutely accept my body as it is today, with my faded stretch marks and sturdy man-sized feet, but I won't accept ever being unhealthy again. Let's face it, if I was to regain weight, not only would I need pants in a bigger size, but I would also struggle to mountain bike up a hill (something I've come to love now). I'd struggle to hike with a pack, to enjoy movement with ease as I do today. I can't even imagine my life today without exercise—it's become such an integral piece of who I am and brings boundless joy. So yes, I accept everything, including the fact that I am choosing to maintain my weight loss, and that requires hard work. Don't most things in life? Certainly those things worth having do.

Ironically, I'm actually a very private person. I'll occasionally post to Instagram, never to Facebook. After all, "Facebook's for old people, Mummy!" exclaimed Emmy.

Perhaps I am old, and is that such a bad thing? No, quite the opposite—it's the ultimate gift, the gift of time, of years with my children. I shall henceforth embrace my age, my wrinkles, and the freedom that comes with maturity and growing wisdom.

Despite my desire for privacy, I realized that this story needed to be told, because it's so much bigger than me (and my former elastic-waisted pants). My experience in the world and the treatment that I received as a size 16 and now a size 6 speaks volumes about the inherent bias that remains for the overweight and obese. And it needs to change, starting with kindness, compassion, and acceptance of different body shapes and sizes. It's true that I wasn't comfortable or happy when overweight, but it's also true that some people are happy. Do we have any right to judge another human? To tell them how they should or shouldn't look? Behave? Dress?

Society is still very open in its discrimination of the overweight and obese. In the workplace and elsewhere we are no longer legally allowed (at least in Canada) to discriminate based upon age, race, gender, or religious affiliation. But if you're fat? Well, look out, because it's open season! And it's deplorable.

As a mother of three beautiful yet impressionable teens, I recognize that the world they are entering is anything but easy to navigate. Yes, the body positivity movement has come a long way, with body acceptance and body neutrality movements gaining traction. Yet when I pull up at the school pickup zone at 3:00 p.m., what I see is sometimes alarming. Girls and boys, some dangerously slender. Many of them see food as a danger, as a vice to be avoided. I'm told by my son that some friends regularly skip meals. It's clear that we still have a long way to go. I don't fear for my own children. I'm reasonably confident that they have learned from my past, my story, and my current healthy behaviors—Lord knows we've discussed it at length! We learn what we live after all, and I see my children now choosing to exercise regularly and cook healthy meals from scratch. All foodies themselves, their smashed-avocado-toast variations put mine to shame, such is their creativity in the kitchen and commitment to wellness.

I fully respect and acknowledge that some people are happy, proud, and comfortable in a larger body, however I was not. I was the opposite of comfortable.

"But Jane, we didn't eat that much!" reasoned Brian recently. "We didn't have a bad diet!"

This was true, but Brian was at work all day. He had no idea if I baked something and ate half of it (on a bad day). How could he? Particularly if I'd frozen the leftovers or made a double recipe.

Despite my physician's warnings about butter and diesel engines post third pregnancy, to this day I still enjoy butter, but I enjoy it in moderation (Apollo, right again). And to be clear, I buy yummy organic grassfed butter, from happy cows—at least happier than those poor feedlot bovines. And after all, it tastes like butter should taste. And I tell myself that if the cows are eating actual green grass, then it's healthier for me, and these free-range beasts have had a better life than their feedlot cousins. It costs more, as healthy food usually does, but I'll save in the long run. Cheap food is a false economy. Cheaper food leads to poor health and increased medical costs—these facts have been well-documented. Healthy food usually leads to greater health and lower medical costs as we age. Win-win.

Surprising was the discovery that I was a threat to people when I started to change—that was interesting. We learn a lot about the people in our world, and fast, when we begin to make dramatic changes in our own lives. It's a curious thing. Some people feel threatened. Why is that? I had some friends (perhaps subconsciously) offer me additional food and wine when I was clearly dieting. (Seriously, did I look like I needed more?!) And why is it upsetting to some when we begin to make positive changes in our own lives? Perhaps because they then feel forced to take a look at their own lives, their health and lifestyles, their daily choices, and habits. I don't doubt that this is the case.

A great deal of my life seems to have been spent feeling judged. Judged as a small child. As a teen. A young adult. A new mother. And everyone judged. My peers. My grandmother. Neighbors. Strangers. The waiter at the restaurant when I'd place my order. Other wives. When my weight would fluctuate. When I left my marriage. Great piles of judgment, bringing to mind the piles of manure that we'd sidestepped on the Camino that spring. And what did I ultimately learn from this never-ending judgment? That it doesn't matter. None of it matters. We can't control a single thing another person thinks, says, or does. Only one person's opinion matters, and that's our own.

As Napoleon Hill wisely advises, "Keep your own counsel."

Indeed.

And why is it that when I enter a dining establishment with a man that I am afforded more respect? Just a little more attention, often a faster table. Yet I could be entering with my children, with the same outfit and attention to my appearance, and I'm given just a little less attention, slightly less respect. Why is that? Our patriarchal society, always at work in the most subtle of ways. It's disgusting. And a less observant person may not even notice, however, having a keen eye for subtle shifts in energy, I notice everything. My fascination with the study of human behavior has only intensified with the passing years. To be fair, Dr. A is six foot four and usually well-dressed, so I suppose he commands respect in the way that only a privileged older white male can, but that doesn't make it okay, does it?

If I sound a little angry, perhaps it's because I am. No one told me this growing up. No one told me that it would be harder to find a rental apartment when I tell them that I'm a single mother (solo parent!). That when I'd head to the auto mall to (finally) buy a car that the salesman would ask me if my husband would be joining us. No, he fucking wouldn't! Does the fact that this question was posed from an older gentleman, clearly born into a different world, make it any less inappropriate? Less offensive? Good Lord. The patriarchy really is alive and flourishing.

The universe does have a sense of humor, and a good one. You see, I used to be something of a snobby homeowner. I'm ashamed to admit that we had some rather, shall we say, colorful neighbors at one time. They were renting; we were in company housing and owned property elsewhere, and I felt superior. I was about twenty-nine years old at the time, and I wish I had known better than to judge. I'm ashamed to write these words, but it's true. You see, their backyard crap could rival my fathers (although theirs was devoid of a forklift), and their multiple children were all out of control, running amok with predictable regularity. And this is saying something because Lord knows mine were a handful.

Their kids were rambunctious, and I learned very quickly that their parents had very different values to ours, and vastly different ideas about what constituted appropriate children's gifts. You see, one pleasant autumn afternoon, their youngest, who was all of five, decided to bring a knife with him to our home after school. Why? Well, apparently, he wanted to impress my children with his birthday gift. In the kitchen at the time, I was preparing after-school snacks for my own offspring and the local kids who lived across the road. Our front lawn, trampoline, and swing set were the site of many a happy afternoon, save this one.

I spotted the knife. It looked sharp, the blade was not covered, and young Ben was excitedly waving it in my direction, evidently with the goal of impressing us all with his weapon.

"Ben, honey, we're going to have to take that home now!" Alarmed but remaining calm (I do possess that gift), I ushered the young chap safely outside and down the pebbled driveway. Thankfully, I convinced Ben that I should hold it on the walk home. To this day he probably thinks I wanted a closer look, after all, that was my reasoning then as I negotiated with young Ben (mercifully this worked at the time).

"Off we go!" My voice was singsong as I instructed my two not to run onto the road, light a fire, etc., while I was gone.

Knocking gently on the front door, I was met by their mother, who looked decidedly more harried than I.

"I thought I told you to keep that in your bedroom!" Ben's father barked from the living room. His bedroom?! To be clear, we are talking about one of those angry-looking, solid, six-inch blades that could kill a man. And Ben was five. And word on the street was that Ben's uncle (who also came and went frequently) had done time, was released, and shouldn't be anywhere near children, given the nature of his reported crimes. It was all rather disturbing really, and I could be forgiven for calling them "the renters." Of course, fast forward to 2024, and I'm the lowly renter. So perhaps I deserve this for my superior attitude all those years back? Is this my karma for being less compassionate in my youth? Mind you, I still don't let my children play with knives. There are limits.

In any event, after finally moving past these judgments (mine and others'), it was time to figure out who I was on my own. I didn't have that period of discovery and exploration in my twenties like most people do. Not until my early forties did I truly find happiness alone, content and complete. Confident, finally. This was the lesson. One of the many, I suppose.

You see, we all grew up together really, Brian and I, navigating our way and guiding the children concurrently. That's the thing about starting a family in our twenties. I gently guided my children—to the best of my abilities—while also growing into the woman I was destined to become.

You may be amused to hear that Sally Newton, of the unfortunate pubic hair debacle, shared her own come-to-Jesus moment years later when she reached out. Regretful of her unkind bullying (and perhaps racist implications toward an entire continent?!), I received quite a touching apology via email and immediately sent up a prayer for Sally and her follicular challenges. As for Amanda Wilson, I have no doubt that she's out there somewhere, stealing hearts and blasting farts. Lord knows, both were her specialties.

obsession

*Somewhere between obsession
and compulsion is impulse.*

—Alexander Pushkin

Binge eating and compulsive shopping.

Turns out it's dangerously easy to slide from one disorder into the other, replacing one compulsive behavior with a different but equally unhelpful pattern of behavior. For many, these are co-occurring. Both are tied to struggles with self-control and impulsivity. Psychology tells us that this is very easy to do. Turns out, far too easy, and I should know. Many years ago, I realized that I had successfully replaced my eating disorder with a compulsive shopping disorder. Now to be fair it was mild, but nevertheless problematic. My commitment to my newfound hobby would have been impressive if it weren't for the fact that I was simply spending too much money.

"You become obsessed with things, Jane. You're obsessive," my mother reminded me.

"Yes, yes, this I know."

We both knew this. Mother was right, as is often the case. Of course, I obsess. I'm a Scorpio. I don't know any other way. It's what we do!

Looking back, I had conveniently replaced one destructive behavior with another. Reasoning that shopping was the lesser of two evils, I'd justify the purchase of a new dress in a heartbeat. From a practical standpoint, it did make sense. My shape was changing, and despite my ex-husband's advice to just "put a belt on," I opted for new jeans. Can you imagine? Down multiple sizes, my old clothing was still mortifying to look at, such was my shame. The only thing that prevented me from burning the lot was the knowledge that someone at a thrift store would benefit, and that burning clothing (or anything, I suppose) is an ecological nightmare for our already stressed planet. My postmarriage budget didn't exactly allow for an unbridled shopping addiction—the numbers just weren't there. A conundrum to be sure, but ever optimistic, I decided that it was time to make some more money. It was either that or give up the Reformation dresses that I'd come to love, and hell would freeze over before I'd allow that to happen.

I'm definitely still working on this challenge. After all, a new pair of jeans is sugar-free! I'm very good at talking myself into any purchase, and I've always had an obsessive personality. Let's not forget the era of all things Sebastian. Historically, I'd never been a fan of moderation—just never very good at it. Be it love, food, or exercise. I'm either all in, or not at all. But I'm learning. Always learning.

And while we're on the subject of shopping, how has it taken me forty-five years to discover the versatility of the humble cargo pants? Pants with useable pockets! Genius. And why, for so long, have pants with large pockets been only the purview of men? Was the patriarchy keeping this from us too? I have to wonder. Now I don't know about anyone else, but I find that the multitude of zippered and buttoned pockets on modern women's cargo pants are incredibly useful. Who knew?! I can now leave the house without a purse. Sure, not every day, but when I actually utilize these pockets for a key/phone/tampon, I can go just about anywhere. Just brilliant. It occurred to me that, given the fickle nature of the fashion industry, I should really stock up on these pants while I can. After all, who knows when they will be no longer in vogue, and I'll be stuck having to carry a purse everywhere again? Now if you'll excuse me, I'm off to the mall.

walk

I am not what happened to me.
I am what I choose to become.

—Carl Jung

I feel that it's very important to reiterate the following: Many people are truly happy in their bodies at a larger weight. Happier in a larger body, loving and embracing their physiques, and I have nothing but admiration and respect for them. This just wasn't my experience. I wasn't comfortable when I was clinically obese. I lacked energy, I was uncomfortable. I'd sweat so easily in summer; my thighs would chafe. I was never truly at ease. There was just too much of me. I ached to buy the current fashions of the day. Well, with the exception of that dreadful revival, culottes. There are limits.

My old school friend Dion shared the following wisdom that I think we'd all do well to remember: "Jane, culottes make you look shorter and wider than you are, and if you ever wear them, I will shoot you!"

Yes, turns out they do, and I have the pregnancy photos to prove it. Fortunately for me, Dion didn't follow through with his threat of death. Just what are designers thinking sometimes? I still don't know.

As for my current appearance, I am now treated with considerably more respect by everyone, and it's incredibly sad. Actually, it's appalling. When I was overweight, I had more money and less respect. Now I have less money and more respect. And why is this? Because of my external appearance, that's why. There is simply no other reason. It's almost laughable—the irony and madness of it all. Yes, I'll concede that I do carry myself with more confidence now, and politely demand respect (and I sure as hell don't wear maternity culottes), but it's more than that. It didn't matter how well dressed I was when I was overweight. Salespeople would still look through me, dismissive. When I'd take the family SUV to the mechanic for that overpriced regular service, I'd usually receive a polite but dismissive reception. The reception now is one of warmth, of appreciation. At a bar ordering drinks, I no longer have to wait. Where doors were once closed, they're now open. It's nothing short of madness and speaks to deeply entrenched biases that remain in society today, where a person's size is equated with morality. I am acutely aware of the thin privilege that I now possess. Also embedded in racism, my now slim white body is seen as the ideal, and it's abhorrent. All of it.

Mine is a unique position to be in. I've experienced walking into a room and being invisible. Ignored by men and women alike, sometimes met with responses that ranged from ambivalence to disdain. I experience the opposite reaction now. Ambivalence by some for sure, but often appreciation now. Current responses range from warmth to approval, sometimes desire. Having navigated the world at both ends of the physically-socially acceptable spectrum, I am in an exceptional situation. I have a heightened awareness of my power as a woman who looks a certain way, yet I also know how it feels to look and be treated in the opposite manner, by both men and women.

Let's be clear—I'm healthy now physically because I'm healthy now mentally. I don't believe the two can be separated, and I certainly don't believe that weight loss can be maintained without doing the emotional work—the excavating, the reckoning, and ultimately healing. The inner work must come first, or concurrently, for long term change to be possible. We can't change the outside without changing the inside, the internal landscape. I know that I certainly couldn't. Until I addressed my deep-seated insecurities and their origins, I couldn't begin to make real change.

Old habits die hard, and it's a case of progress, not perfection. There are still days I'll slide, falling back into old habits at lightning speed. And then I catch myself, and I remember, self-compassion! So dearly lacking for so long. I'm still working on self-compassion, self-love, on forgiveness when those few pounds creep on—and then I make an active and very conscious choice to drop them. It's not easy, but it's a choice, a choice to maintain my health. And it's hard work. The legacy of my former body, mine is an extremely efficient fat-cell-producing machine.

I've also had to separate my desire to remain healthy from any pressure to look a certain way for a man. These are loaded feelings, and I'm still working to reconcile this complex web of emotions. My health and wellness versus external pressure to conform. Despite our progress as a society, I don't forget the ways in which I was treated so poorly by the outside world when I was overweight. What does this say of our society? Why are we still allowed to discriminate against the obese so overtly? I was the same person beneath my skin. We all are, irrespective of our changing external appearances.

Rainn Wilson tells us that we are spiritual beings having a human experience, and I wholeheartedly agree. Dwight is right! (And he's also right about beets, they really are delicious.) Our body is a vessel, and the only one that we have on this exhilarating ride for eighty plus years if we're lucky. I've chosen to love mine, with gratitude for its capabilities. I choose to nurture with good food, movement that brings joy, and a glass of red or two when I wish. Restriction doesn't work and prohibition is madness. What we forbid, we desire—I learned that early on. If I feel like baking cookies, I'll bake them. Only now I'll have one, not the five or six in a day that would have led to physical discomfort, guilt, disgust, regret, and shame. Ahh, the good old days. Now I'm hungry for the outdoors, for foreign lands. Hungry to try a new Instagram salad recipe. Hungry for adventure, for new experiences. Hungry for life.

As a child, I ached to be exploring. Growing up on an isolated, remote island continent, I wonder if our collective isolation is why many Australians feel this wanderlust? This desire to breach our shores and discover the broad, wide world beyond. I certainly did, and now I find myself making up for lost time. Looking back, I took on so much responsibility at such a young age; I don't recommend it. Perhaps on a very subconscious level, I knew this all along, my yearning to travel and explore dormant, deep within the recesses of my soul, waiting to be awakened. I hungered for a freedom that would be decades incoming.

I now move every day. I walk, hike, or bike daily, doing something to nurture my body. And not everybody likes exercise, and I completely respect that. For me, exercise remains cathartic. I sweat and feel better, honoring my body in the process. Maintenance requires movement; it's simply nonnegotiable. A tired day means yoga or a walk. Something to ensure that I connect with my body on a visceral level. Interoceptive awareness is also essential to maintenance.

Walking past someone very overweight earlier today on my morning constitutional, I smiled. They met my gaze, looking just slightly apologetic and uncomfortable; my heart went out to them. I knew that look, that feeling of inadequacy; it was mine a decade prior.

"That doesn't even look like you!" But it was. Isabelle couldn't hide her surprise, her eyes widened, as I reluctantly shared a "before" photo. She'd never seen me at my heaviest, having shed quite a bit of baby weight before emigrating to Canada eleven years prior. These were also the days before social media truly took over our world, and this afforded me a unique opportunity to hide. To conceal. No one need ever know of my dirty, shameful secret. After all, I'd moved to the north shore of Vancouver, home of the most eating disorders in Canada, and a disproportionate number of women in tight yoga pants, with their perfect thighs, perfect houses, and perfect husbands. It was dangerous. Comparisons are never helpful, and filled with self-loathing for my past, I chose not to share my prior struggles. After all, I reasoned, I was still in the process of losing the rest of the weight. Why did anyone need to know just how enormous I'd been at one time? For the most part, my fat days were in the pre-social media days, and I was grateful that none of these pictures were easily found.

Again, there is a God.

Owning this reality now is essential to my healing, to truly make peace with my past. Am I 100 percent there? No, but I'm trying. I'm close. And this book has become instrumental in reconciling the past with the present.

fat cells

Be grateful for your difficulties and challenges,
for they hold blessings. In fact . . . Man needs
difficulties; they are necessary for health, personal
growth, individuation, and self-actualisation.

—Carl Jung

Apparently, as humans, we renew every cell in our body every seven years. And our bones every ten years! While there may be some debate as to this exact length of time, I've come to the conclusion that my body is entirely new at this point. I am essentially a new person. Wow.

Am I still the girl who built herself a homemade swimming pool in the backyard because her parents couldn't afford one? Yes. The girl who had to shop in the plus-size section of the department store? Yes. I need to own this, and I need to own it because I didn't want to. I haven't wanted to for the past decade. And it's time to own it. It still feels a little humiliating to write these words. It was sure as hell humiliating at the time.

I recall postpregnancy clothes shopping in the early 2000s—choice was limited, and bloody ugly offerings, let me tell you. Why the fuck did designers think that overweight women want to adorn their bodies in huge swathes of lurid patterned, synthetic fabrics? I appreciate that times have changed, as they should, and thank goodness. But I also know that when I had to shop in the plus-size section of the store, it was nothing short of traumatizing. Without a doubt, that was a contributing factor in my motivation, my determination to transform my body. Transforming my life came later. But my appearance was one of frustration. I ached to walk into any store and buy anything I loved in a regular size. I love to shop for beautiful clothes now, despite my champagne taste and prosecco budget. Definitely still working to reconcile this one.

At a recent checkup with the handsome surgeon, Dr. S found what he delicately termed "a small pocket of fat." Horrified, I examined my stomach from multiple angles. Those persistent little fuckers! Fat cells! Who knew they'd be so impatient to come back at the slightest opportunity? For a brief moment I had something of a come-to-Jesus moment of my own. I realized then, and know now, that vigilance is required if I wish to maintain my new physique. It's a fact of life. The sky is blue, and I must work at maintenance. And work hard. It's a choice and my reality.

"Do you know how many people lose the kind of weight that you've lost and keep it off, Jane? Have a guess."

"Umm, I know it's a small number," saying as I stood half-naked in front of my lovely surgeon.

He looked at me. "Two percent."

That hit me, as did his praise that I try and accept with humility.

"Women are so hard on themselves!" he mused, and I knew he was telling me to be kinder to myself, as I stared, always critical in his full-length mirror. The bright lights never forgiving, leaving nothing to the imagination. My stretch marks were fading with the passage of time, as was the surgical scar. My tummy scar barely visible now, the surgery done so well in the first place, it was always hidden neatly below my bikini bottoms. Yet more to add to my gratitude list!

"The magic that you are looking for is in the work that you are avoiding."

Now, while I can't be credited with coining this phrase, I do wish to share it here. It's currently raining outside, and my hair is still wet from my recent shower. As I type this, I realize that seeing this quote today on my Instagram feed was the reminder that I needed to lace up my hiking boots and get a workout in, despite the lousy weather. Did I want to head out into the cold when I was cozy, sitting up in bed, enjoying my morning espresso and catching up on texts that came in from Australia while I slept? No, I didn't. But did I find the magic outside when I choose not to avoid the work? Hell yes.

I always do.

I recently learned that our brains actually clear out toxins when we exercise! (Thank you, Dr. A, for this brief lesson.) The cognitive benefits are well-documented now, and I can feel them as I type with increased clarity and appreciation for my body. Yes, life is work. And fortunately, also play! And I have to say that once I'm outside on the mountain, it begins to feel more like play than work. Then again, so did time with Javier, and that certainly wasn't outdoors, but I digress.

Dr. Giles Yeo, author of *Why Calories Don't Count*, tells us that exercise is very good for weight maintenance. Not so much for weight loss, as we can't outrun a bad diet. I've found this to be accurate overall. Dr. Yeo also makes the point that exercise makes us hungrier, hence the need for restraint post-workout. And it's not always easy. Some days it's still hard, but it's achievable. It really is. I think almost anything is, if we want it badly enough. And perhaps that's the key—we have to want it badly enough, so badly that we are prepared to make short-term sacrifices in order to achieve our goal of fat loss.

Intermittent fasting. Increasing in popularity, I want to touch on my experiences with this type of routine here. I do feel the benefits of intermittent fasting, and I find that there's a mental clarity that arises when I give my digestion a break. There is, however, one huge caveat that I must mention: You must be able to resume moderate, healthy eating upon breaking the fast. Ending a fast and overconsuming to make up for everything missed, well, that just puts one right back where they started. Not a good idea. Personally, I do find a sixteen-hour/eight-hour pattern of eating quite natural some days and will sometimes eat this way without any restriction or use of will on my part.

Essentially, on these days I'll enjoy coffee for breakfast, eat lunch at noon, afternoon tea, followed by a meal in the evening. When 8:00 p.m. comes around some days, I find myself completely satiated and not hungry in the slightest. And if I've eaten a large dinner, I'm often not hungry until lunchtime the following day anyway, so in some ways it's been quite natural to adopt this pattern of eating from time to time. It's not for everybody, however (much like Nebraska), and I merely share here what I have found that works for me some days after a decade at a healthy, stable weight. And if I want breakfast, feeling true hunger, then of course I'll have it. Deprivation doesn't work. First and foremost, I listen to my body's internal hunger cues, because my body knows exactly what it needs. And if I am physically hungry, I eat, mindful to choose nourishing whole foods whenever possible.

As it happened, I had additional time to practice mindfulness techniques. Boarding a painfully long economy flight, intermittent fasting was preferable to eating whatever crap the good airline decided to surprised me with. This meal was memorable for all the wrong reasons. You see, I had to go home. My sister, having been airlifted to Melbourne from my mother's small country town, was in the hospital. No longer could I avoid that God-awful fifteen-hour Vancouver–Brisbane leg that would effectively connect me with my family in rural Victoria, Australia. I'm also aware that, as the family member not in hospital, complaining about my cramped economy seat really is something of a champagne problem. After all, I'm grateful and fortunate to be able to buy the ticket, visit with my sister, and help my long-suffering mother (even if I can hear my credit card audibly groaning under the weight of recent purchases).

So, I'd boarded, it was 1:30 a.m., and our flight was delayed due to volcanic ash over the Pacific. Evidently there's a volcano in Russia spewing ash all over the planet. I immediately concluded that if there's one place that any form of eating restriction goes out the window, it's at forty-thousand feet. *Now is not the time to fast.* I did come prepared with emergency pistachios packed into a reusable container. As for the environmental benefit, my eco-warrior vegan eldest wholeheartedly approved. I was saving the planet one protein-filled snack at a time! (Mind you, I really should have also packed an almond croissant—what was I was thinking?)

It's been six years since I've set foot on Australian soil. Away too long, but in that time, there was a divorce, a pandemic, grad school. Stuff happened. Life happened. Stepping into the terminal in Brisbane just felt wonderful—it's impossible to explain or quantify. And everyone sounded just like me, only more so.

Happy tears.

love

Courage is knowing what not to fear.

—Plato

s I write these words, I realize that I have nothing to fear. My initial fears when penning this memoir were of revealing the well-buried secret of my weight gain and loss. So much fear. Fear of not being loveable. Of being found unattractive, as I was deemed by many people when my pants were a far bigger size.

And then it hit me. Love isn't conditional. If it's conditional, then it isn't love. And with this realization comes the knowledge that I have nothing to fear. Those who truly love me will continue to do so, and I them. If someone from my new world reads these words and takes exception to my former size, well then, they never truly loved me anyway.

This book is therefore something of an experiment. It shall weed out the insincere in my life. How wonderful. Really, this is a potential time saver! If someone in my world does love me conditionally, I'd rather know about it now. Imagine finding out in the future that a friend or lover who proclaimed to love me only does so for who I am now, conditionally, in my socially acceptable size 6 body? And if that is the case, then this book has done me a monumental favor, saving me the time of discovering this knowledge at a later date.

I have nothing to fear.

Perhaps it's even time to be proud of the work I put into losing the weight. Why haven't I been proud of this? Too much shame over gaining it in the first place, I suppose. This needed to change. And through publishing this book and sharing my deepest secrets with anyone who has a desire to pick this up in a bookstore, I hope to make peace with my past. Shame no longer has any place in my new world.

The most wonderful thing about being in one's forties is that I just don't care anymore. I refer, of course, to other people's opinions. Don't care. After all, we're all going to die. Imagine living with constant fear and angst, obsessing over what another human being may or may not think about us? What an utter waste of a lifetime! I refuse to allow fear to ever dictate a decision, refuse to allow my thoughts, actions, or behaviors to be hijacked by it.

What I do care about is kindness. If we could all just be kind to each other from birth until death, well, how very lovely the world could be. It's so simple really. Kind irrespective of our physical appearance, devoid of judgment. Kind because, as members of the human race, we deserve nothing less. Kind because, like it or not, we all share this planet together for a brief moment in time. Why does it remain so difficult for some people to extend kindness? Humanity to another human? I think I know why, and it's because some people carry pain, and aren't as far along on their journey, and I accept that. Again, acceptance.

In Spain we found kindness on the Camino. Weary pilgrims would happily share advice, a warm *"Buen Camino,"* suggestions for accommodation, or where to find the best food. In these moments, somewhere along that trail, I looked at my two younger children, fearlessly marching along beside me, and realized that I had found what I'd been searching for. Love.

I found it on the trail with my children. Their laughter, the warmth of the early spring sunshine, our shared joy at the spectacular, idyllic countryside. Hungry for life, for adventure, I was finally satiated. My heart swelled with love and gratitude.

Happy tears.

I know that I will write for the rest of my days, sharing my humble thoughts with anyone who wishes to read them. Writing led to answers, helping me to distill and clarify my thoughts. Writing invariably leads to solutions. The truth. Writing this memoir has led me to the truth of who I am, what I want, and where I want to go in this next stage of my life. What I need and don't need (this is a big one).

The whole process has been rather useful in hindsight!

Sinking into my mother's soft leather couch, I realized that this brief time in Australia facilitated reflection. Physical distance begets mental clarity. It feels appropriate that I needed to return home to come full circle, making peace with my past. And then I was gone again, returning to my new Vancouver home.

There's excitement too, for the future. It comes in waves. And determination. Determination to take every opportunity to explore our broad wide world, continuing to grow and better myself.

Hungry for life. Always.

My favorite song also contains my favorite lines. The brilliant, underrated country singer, Cody Jinks, penned the following:

"Loud thunder, heavy rain
Thin line 'tween joy and pain
It's a long strange trip, it's all insane
You ain't never gonna be the same."

He's singing my life. It is all insane. And beautiful. And for all the joy, equal measures of pain. And I wouldn't trade this long, strange trip for anything.

My eyes fill with tears of gratitude and love when I check on my sleeping children. Not children anymore, my eldest now twenty. All three of my precious, nearly grown children are under my roof and sleeping peacefully while the snow falls gently outside. For once Vancouver is quiet. And in this moment, I know that I'm luckier and more blessed than I have any right to be, and I say a prayer to the universe for every day that we have together. *Thank you.*

Acknowledgments

As I sit here and begin this, it occurs to me that everyone who has ever crossed my path in the last forty-seven years has contributed in some way to my growth as I evolved into the woman that I am today. The woman who was able to write this book in three sleep-deprived, caffeine-fueled, laugh-out-loud months. I am therefore grateful to everyone!

Now, I appreciate that this is a rather broad statement, and it would be remiss of me not to mention many of the beautiful souls whom I am blessed to love. I'm not sure what I did to deserve such wonderful humans in my life, but I'll take it! Your ongoing love and support remains invaluable, and continues to allow me to pursue this new career with relentless determination. Thank you!

To my long-suffering mother, Jan, I owe everything. I still don't know how you had the patience to withstand the last few decades and retain your smile and sense of humor, but you did. This speaks to your strength, which I remain grateful to have inherited (at least in part). We really are a resilient bunch!

To my sister, Fi, I love you dearly (despite not demonstrating this often). And yes, I know I was a crap sister at times.

To my Core (Pour/Poor) Four, I love you all so much!! Kellie, Mar, Tiff, and Tom (alphabetized, FYI): Thank you for your love, laughter, and friendship with the crazy Australian. Please know that you are stuck with me forever.

To my ex-husband, thank you for our three phenomenal children and for the good years that we shared before it all went to hell.

To Dr. A, thank you for teaching me to mountain bike!

To Brooke Warner and her team, for loving my crazy manuscript and taking a chance on this unpublished (and very new to the game) author—thank you!

Also, thank you to Chuck, for your invaluable assistance early on in this publication process!

Above all, to my children—CB, Emily, and Alex. You are my life, my world, and my three greatest joys. I love you more than you can know (and thank you for your patience when Mummy talked about her book!).

There is a tangible ache in my chest as I type these words. A good ache. It's visceral, this love, entwined with gratitude, with joy and excitement for tomorrow, for adventures yet unknown. And I wonder, what did I ever do to deserve the three most incredible humans on the planet?

I still don't know.

About the Author

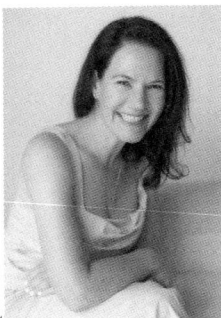

Jane McGuinness is a Registered Clinical Counsellor and mother of three fearless young Australians. A recovering emotional eater, her own therapy consists of escaping to the mountains whenever possible to hike or bike with her trademark enthusiasm for life. North Vancouver is currently home for this Aussie expat who advocates acceptance, gratitude, and kindness above all else, and maintains that a day without laughter is a day wasted.

Looking for your next great read?

We can help!

Visit www.shewritespress.com/next-read
or scan the QR code below for a list
of our recommended titles.

She Writes Press is an award-winning
independent publishing company founded to
serve women writers everywhere.

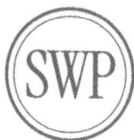